Heart Failure

an

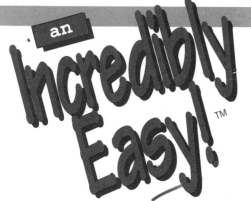

Incredibly Easy!™

MiniGuide

Heart Failure

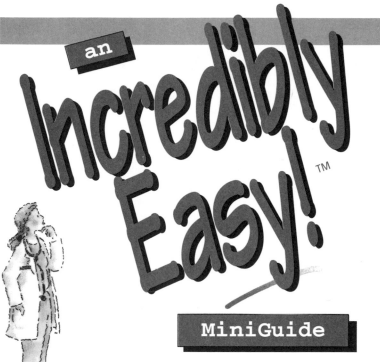

an

Incredibly Easy! ™

MiniGuide

Springhouse Corporation
Springhouse, Pennsylvania

Staff

Vice President
Matthew Cahill

Clinical Director
Judith A. Schilling McCann, RN, MSN

Art Director
John Hubbard

Executive Editor
Michael Shaw

Managing Editor
Andrew T. McPhee, RN, BSN

Clinical Editors
Jill Curry, RN, BSN, CCRN; Carla M. Roy, RN, BSN, CCRN; Joan M. Robinson, RN, MSN, CCRN

Editors
Christine Adamec, Serita Stevens, Patricia Wittig

Copy Editors
Brenna H. Mayer (manager), Mary T. Durkin, Gretchen Fee, Stacey Ann Follin, Pamela Wingrod

Designers
Arlene Putterman (associate art director), Mary Ludwicki (book designer), Joseph Clark, Jacalyn B. Facciolo

Illustrators
Bot Roda, Betty Winnberg, Jacalyn B. Facciolo

Typography
Diane Paluba (manager), Joyce Rossi Biletz, Valerie Molettiere

Manufacturing
Deborah Meiris (director), Patricia K. Dorshaw (manager), Otto Mezei (book production manager)

Editorial Assistants
Beverly Lane, Marcia Mills, Liz Schaeffer

Indexer
Ellen Murray

Printed in the United States of America.

IEMHF-010899

® A member of the Reed Elsevier plc group

Library of Congress Cataloging-in-Publication Data

Heart failure: an incredibly easy miniguide
    p. cm. (Incredibly easy miniguide)
    Includes index.
    ISBN 1-58255-011-5 (alk. paper)
    1. Heart failure Handbooks, manuals, etc. 2. Heart failure—Nursing handbooks, manuals, etc.
    I. Springhouse Corporation.
    II. Series
[DNLM: 1. Heart failure, Congestive Handbooks.
WG 39 H4357 1999]
RC685.C53H825 1999
616.1'29—dc21
DNLM/DLC
99-25002
                        CIP

Contents

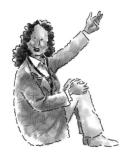

Contributors and consultants

Joanne M. Bartelmo, RN, MSN, CCRN
Clinical Educator
Pottstown (Pa.) Memorial
Medical Center

Nancy Cirone, RN,C, MSN, CDE
Director of Education
Warminster (Pa.) Hospital

Margaret Friant Cramer, RN, MSN
Clinical Supervisor
Cardiac Solutions, Inc.
Fort Washington, Pa.

Pamela Mullen Kovach, RN, BSN
Independent Clinical
Consultant
Perkiomenville, Pa.

Patricia A. Lange, RN, MSN, EdD, CS, CCRN
Graduate Nursing Program
Coordinator and Assistant
Professor of Nursing
Hawaii Pacific University
Kaneohe

Mary Ann Siciliano McLaughlin, RN, MSN
Clinical Supervisor
Cardiac Solutions, Inc.
Fort Washington, Pa.

Lori Musolf Neri, RN, MSN, CCRN
Clinical Instructor
Villanova (Pa.) University
ICU Staff Nurse
North Penn Hospital
Lansdale, Pa.

Joseph L. Neri, DO, FACC
Cardiologist
The Heart Care Group
Allentown, Pa.

Robert Rauch
Manager of Government
Economics
Amgen, Inc.
Thousand Oaks, Calif.

Larry E. Simmons, RN, PhD
Clinical Instructor
University of Missouri-
Kansas City

Foreword

Each year, health care professionals in the United States care for nearly 5 million patients with heart failure. Many of these patients also have diabetes, hypertension, or any of a wide variety of other ailments.

Meeting the challenges of caring for a patient with heart failure requires a full understanding of the disorder and its implications for care. At once accurate, authoritative, and completely up-to-date, this handy book can help you gain an in-depth understanding of heart failure in an amazingly fun and exciting way.

The first chapter, Understanding heart failure, lays the foundation for your understanding by providing basic facts about the pathophysiology of heart failure and the effects of heart failure on the body. The next three chapters cover prevention, assessment, and treatment for heart failure. The fifth chapter covers complications of the disorder, and the final chapter covers patient teaching.

Throughout the book, you'll find features designed to make learning about heart failure lively and entertaining. For instance, *Memory joggers* provide clever tricks for remembering key points. *Checklists,* rendered in the style of a classroom chalkboard, provide at-a-glance summaries of important facts.

Cartoon characters that nearly pop off the page provide light-hearted chuckles as well as reinforcement of essential material. A *Quick quiz* at the end of every chapter gives you a chance to assess your learning and refresh your memory at the same time.

The depth of information contained in this truly pocket-size guide will impress even the most experienced health care professional. If you want a quick-learn, comprehensive reference about one of the most common conditions encountered in health care, I can't think of a more fitting resource than *Heart Failure: An Incredibly Easy MiniGuide.* It packs a wallop.

Michael Carter, RN, DNSc, FAAN
Dean and Professor
College of Nursing
University of Tennessee
Memphis

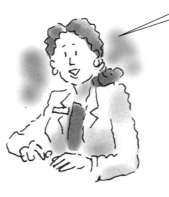

Professional development that's fun and exciting? Incredible!

Understanding heart failure

Key facts
- Heart failure can involve failure of the right side of the heart, the left side, or both.
- Heart failure results from conditions that cause poor ventricular filling or from any condition that limits the heart's ability to pump effectively.
- The body can make short- or long-term adaptations to heart failure.

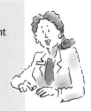

What is heart failure?

Nearly 5 million people in the United States suffer from heart failure. In fact, heart failure is the most common discharge diagnosis for patients over age 65.

Heart failure is not a disease, but a syndrome in which the heart lacks the ability to pump well enough to meet the body's needs. Sometimes the left side of the heart fails; sometimes, the right. (See *A close look at the heart,* page 2.)

A close look at the heart

To refresh your memory of critical heart structures, check this illustration, which shows internal structures of the heart.

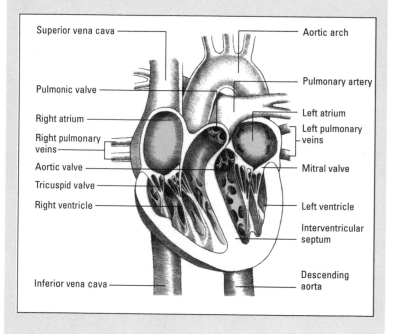

Typically, the left side fails first because the left ventricle pushes blood against greater resistance than the right ventricle.

Certain conditions make it more likely that a patient may develop heart failure. These conditions include:

- arrhythmia
- coronary artery disease
- diabetes mellitus
- pregnancy and thyrotoxicosis, which together increase cardiac output
- pulmonary embolism, which can cause right-sided heart failure
- infection, which can increase metabolic demands
- anemia, which leads to increased cardiac output and a greater workload on the heart because the tissues need more oxygen
- rheumatic heart disease and other forms of myocarditis
- systemic hypertension
- myocardial infarction (MI)
- increased physical activity
- increased salt or water intake
- emotional stress
- failure to comply with the prescribed treatment regimen for underlying heart disease.

Normal heart structure and function

To fully understand heart failure, you need to understand the structure and function of a healthy adult heart.

Step into my chambers

The heart consists of four separate chambers, two atria and two ventricles. The atria are thin-walled chambers that serve as reservoirs for blood. The ventricles have thick walls and are responsible for pumping blood throughout the body.

Blood vessels

Blood is carried into and out of the heart through several major vessels, all of which empty into either the superior vena cava or inferior vena cava. The superior vena cava carries blood from the upper body to the right atrium. The inferior vena cava carries blood from the lower body to the right atrium.

From the atrium to the cardiac interior

Blood in the right atrium empties into the right ventricle mostly by gravity. The blood is then ejected into the pulmonary artery when the ventricle contracts. The blood is pushed through the pulmonary arteries to the lungs.

Now for the final trip through

From the lungs, blood travels to the left atrium through the pulmonary veins. The left atrium empties blood into the left ventricle. The left ventricle pumps the blood into the aorta and from there, throughout the body.

Heart valves

The heart contains two atrioventricular valves (tricuspid and mitral) and two semilunar valves (pulmonic and aortic):

• The tricuspid valve separates the right atrium from the right ventricle.

• The pulmonic valve separates the right ventricle from the pulmonary artery.

• The mitral valve separates the left atrium from the left ventricle.

• The aortic valve separates the left ventricle from the aorta.

Valves in the heart keep blood flowing in one direction. When pressure within a chamber rises past a certain point, the outlet valve opens and the inlet valve closes. For instance, when pressure within the

My four valves — the tricuspid, pulmonic, mitral, and aortic — keep blood moving.

right ventricle reaches a certain point, the tricuspid valve closes and the pulmonic valve opens.

Cardiac cycle

No discussion of heart functions would be complete without an explanation of the cardiac cycle, the period from the beginning of one heartbeat to the beginning of the next. During this cycle, electrical and mechanical events must occur in the proper sequence and to the proper degree to provide adequate blood flow to all body parts. The cardiac cycle has two phases: systole and diastole.

It's systole, not Sister Lee

At the beginning of systole, the ventricles contract, increasing pressure and forcing the mitral and tricuspid valves to close.

Memory jogger

Blood flows through the cardiac valves in this order: tricuspid, pulmonic, mitral, and aortic. But the first letters of these valves — TPMA — occur in *reverse* order in the alphabet. So think: blood flows in reverse alphabetical order. Or remember the mnemonic *Tell Pop the Mail Arrived.*

This closing prevents blood from flowing backward into the atria and coincides with the first heart sound, known as S_1 (the *lub* of the *lub-dub*).

As the ventricles contract, ventricular pressure builds until it exceeds the pressure in the pulmonary artery and aorta. Then the aortic and pulmonic semilunar valves open, and the ventricles eject blood.

It's Diastole, James Diastole

When the ventricles empty and relax, ventricular pressure falls below that in the pulmonary artery and aorta. At the beginning of diastole, the semilunar valves close to prevent the backflow of blood into the ventricles. This action coincides with the second heart sound, known as S_2 (the *dub* of *lub-dub*).

Cardiac output

Cardiac output refers to the amount of blood pumped out by the heart in 1 minute and is determined by the stroke volume, the amount of blood ejected with each heartbeat multiplied by the number of beats per minute. Stroke volume, in

Systole. Diastole. Systole. Diastole. Hey, am I good or what!

turn, depends on three factors: contractility, preload, and afterload.

• *Contractility* refers to the ability of the myocardium to contract normally.

• *Preload* is the stretching of muscle fibers in the ventricles. This stretching results from blood volume in the ventricles at the end of diastole. The more the muscles stretch, the more forcefully they contract during systole.

• *Afterload* refers to the pressure the ventricular muscles must generate to overcome the higher pressure in the aorta. Normally, pressure at the end of diastole (end-diastolic pressure) in the left ventricle measures 5 to 10 mm Hg; in the aorta, it measures 70 to 80 mm Hg.

Pathophysiology

Heart failure may result from any abnormality of the heart muscle that impairs ventricular function and prevents the heart from pumping enough blood. (See *Understanding left- and right-sided heart failure.*) For example, MI can lead to heart failure, particularly if the infarction is severe.

(Text continues on page 17.)

Now I get it!

Understanding left- and right-sided heart failure

The illustrations on these pages show how myocardial damage leads to either left- or right-sided heart failure.

Left-sided heart failure

Increased workload on the heart and an increased blood volume at the end of diastole lead to an enlargement of the left ventricle. (See illustration below.) The patient may experience increased heart rate, pale and cool skin, tingling in the extremities, decreased cardiac output, and arrhythmia.

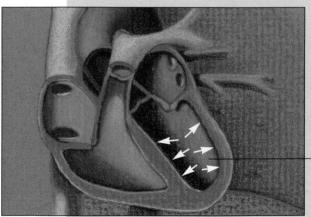

Increased workload enlarges the left ventricle.

(continued)

Understanding left- and right-sided heart failure *(continued)*

Poor left ventricular function allows blood to pool in the ventricle and atrium. Eventually the blood backs into the pulmonary veins and capillaries. (See illustration below.) At this stage, the patient may experience dyspnea on exertion, confusion, dizziness, postural hypotension, decreased peripheral pulses and pulse pressure, cyanosis, and an S_3 gallop.

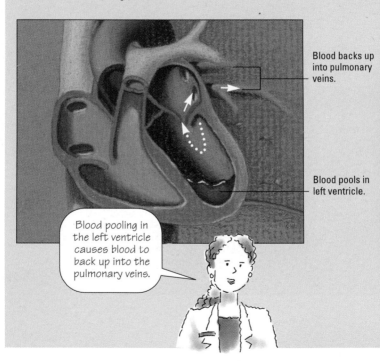

Blood backs up into pulmonary veins.

Blood pools in left ventricle.

Blood pooling in the left ventricle causes blood to back up into the pulmonary veins.

Understanding left- and right-sided heart failure *(continued)*

As pulmonary circulation becomes engorged, capillary pressure increases and pushes sodium and water into interstitial spaces. (See illustration below.) The increase in fluid in the interstitium causes pulmonary edema. You'll note coughing, subclavian retractions, crackles, tachypnea, elevated pulmonary artery pressure, diminished pulmonary compliance, and increased partial pressure of carbon dioxide.

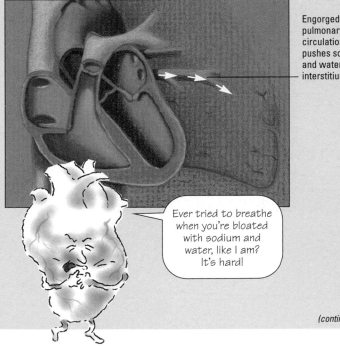

Engorged pulmonary circulation pushes sodium and water into interstitium.

Ever tried to breathe when you're bloated with sodium and water, like I am? It's hard!

(continued)

Understanding left- and right-sided heart failure *(continued)*

When the patient lies down, fluid in the extremities moves into the systemic circulation and eventually reaches the right atrium of the heart. (See illustration below.) Because the left ventricle can't handle the increased venous return, blood pools in the pulmonary circulation, worsening pulmonary edema. You may note decreased breath sounds, dullness on percussion, crackles, and orthopnea.

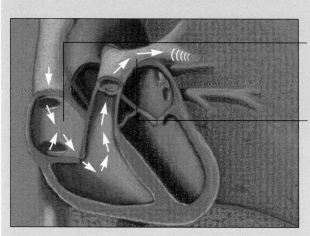

Blood return to the right atrium increases.

Blood pools in the pulmonary circulation.

With a weak left ventricle, I can't keep blood from pooling in the pulmonary circulation. Sorry, lungs!

Understanding left- and right-sided heart failure *(continued)*

The right ventricle, now pumping against greater pulmonary vascular resistance and left ventricular pressure, may become stressed. (See illustration below.) When this occurs, the patient's symptoms worsen.

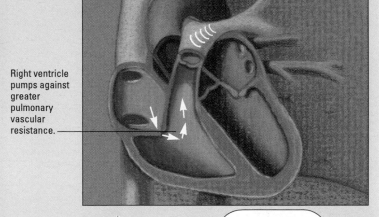

Right ventricle pumps against greater pulmonary vascular resistance.

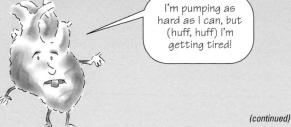

(continued)

Understanding left- and right-sided heart failure *(continued)*

Right-sided heart failure

Stress on the right ventricle causes tissue stretching and ventricular wall enlargement. (See illustration below.) Stretching of myocardial tissue leads to increased conduction time. The increased conduction time, coupled with deviation of the heart from its normal axis, can cause arrhythmia. If the patient doesn't already have left-sided heart failure, he may experience increased heart rate, cool skin, cyanosis, decreased cardiac output, palpitations, and dyspnea.

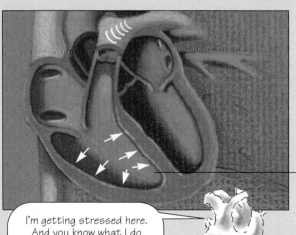

Right ventricular stress leads to tissue stretching and myocardial enlargement.

I'm getting stressed here. And you know what I do when I get stressed? I stretch, twist, and strain.

Understanding left- and right-sided heart failure *(continued)*

Blood pools in the right ventricle and, eventually, the right atrium. The backed-up blood causes pressure and congestion in the venae cavae and systemic circulation. (See illustration below.) Look for elevated central venous pressure, jugular vein distention, and hepatojugular reflux.

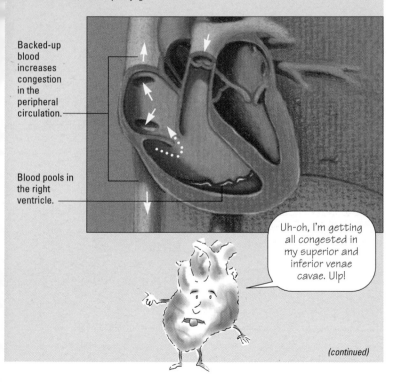

Backed-up blood increases congestion in the peripheral circulation.

Blood pools in the right ventricle.

(continued)

Understanding left- and right-sided heart failure *(continued)*

An increase in capillary pressure forces excess fluid from the capillaries into the interstitial spaces. (See illustration below.) This causes tissue edema, especially in the lower extremities and abdomen. The patient may experience weight gain, pitting edema, and nocturia.

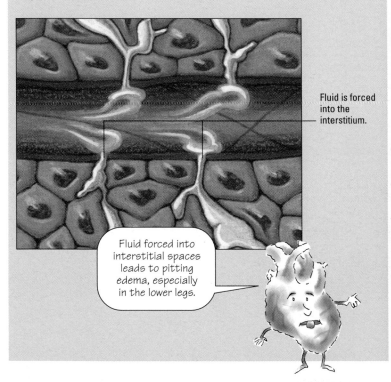

Fluid is forced into the interstitium.

Fluid forced into interstitial spaces leads to pitting edema, especially in the lower legs.

Heart failure may result from poor ventricular filling, which occurs when the volume of circulating blood is too low for the ventricles to pump efficiently.

The heart can also fail as a result of any systolic disturbance that limits the heart's pumping ability or reduces resistance in systemic blood vessels. Systolic disturbances can be caused by volume overload or excessive vessel pressure.

Forms of heart failure

Heart failure can be classified as right- or left-sided heart failure, forward or backward heart failure, acute or chronic heart failure, or low- or high-output heart failure. Let's look at each form.

Right-sided...

Right-sided heart failure occurs when the ability of the right ventricle to contract is impaired and, as a result, rendered ineffective. This variation of heart failure may result from acute right ventricular MI or, possibly, pulmonary embolus.

Uh-oh. If I don't have enough blood to pump, I'm likely to fail.

...or left-sided

Left-sided heart failure occurs most often and usually results from profound back-flow of blood into the left ventricle. Blood backs up in this chamber as a result of poor left ventricular function.

As the pumping ability of the left ventricle decreases, blood isn't fully pumped out of the left ventricle. Eventually, the accumulated blood prevents all the blood in the atrium from flowing into the ventricle. As the atrium keeps receiving blood from the pulmonary veins, it fills up and causes blood to back up into the pulmonary veins and, eventually, into the lungs, causing pulmonary edema. Without treatment, blood will back up into the right ventricle and then the right atrium, causing right-sided heart failure.

Left-sided causes

Common causes of left-sided heart failure include:
• aortic or mitral valve stenosis or regurgitation
• hypertension
• left ventricular MI.

Forward...

Forward heart failure is caused by increased peripheral vascular resistance, or afterload. In hypertension and certain other conditions, afterload is increased and the heart must work harder to pump blood against the increased resistance. That resistance puts a greater workload on the heart.

When the afterload increases, the left ventricle can't eject as much blood as it usually can. Less blood being ejected results in decreased blood flow to and perfusion of vital organs.

Increased afterload and the forward heart failure that may result are usually caused by hypertension or aortic stenosis.

> Severe backward heart failure can cause blood to back up into the lungs and can result in right-sided heart failure.

...or backward

Backward heart failure results when the left ventricle fails to empty completely. The leftover blood causes fluid to accumulate in the left ventricle and the lungs. If fluid congestion in the lungs is severe enough, backward heart failure can lead to right-sided heart failure.

Backward heart failure is usually associated with MI and cardiomyopathy.

Acute...

In acute heart failure, signs and symptoms of failure are new, and compensatory mechanisms — such as natural diuresis — haven't yet kicked in. Typically, the amount of circulating fluid is at a normal level or is low, and sodium and water retention haven't yet occurred.

...or chronic

In chronic heart failure, signs and symptoms of failure have been present for an extended period, and compensatory mechanisms have taken effect. Fluid volume is increased.

Low ventricular output...

Heart failure can also be related to low ventricular output. In MI, hypotension, cardiomyopathy, or hemorrhage, the left ventricle may not be able to eject normal quantities of blood to the vital organs.

Heart failure can result from MI, hypotension, and other conditions in which ventricular output is low.

...or high ventricular output

Conversely, certain conditions that elevate ventricular output can lead to heart failure. Such conditions include pregnancy, thyrotoxicosis, and anemia.

How the heart responds

As stress on the heart muscle increases, the heart muscle's ability to contract is reduced and cardiac output declines. Blood flow into the ventricles usually remains the same, however.

Making some adjustments

Without the ability to eject normal amounts of blood, the ventricles begin to accumulate blood. As the amount of blood in the ventricles increases, the heart makes both short- and long-term adaptations:

• *Short-term adaptations*. The accumulation of blood in the ventricles causes ventricular muscle fibers to increase in length at the end of diastole. As end-diastolic fiber length increases, the muscles re-

> As heart failure persists, my muscles contract less and my output declines. Sure I still pump, but not as well.

spond by dilating and increasing the force of contraction, an occurrence described by the Frank-Starling Law.

• *Long-term adaptations.* If heart failure continues long enough, ventricular hypertrophy occurs. In ventricular hypertrophy, the myocardium enlarges, which in turn increases the heart's ability to push blood into the circulation. Ventricular hypertrophy can adequately compensate for heart failure for a time, but eventually the heart muscle weakens and acute failure ensues.

Quick quiz

1. The left side of the heart tends to fail sooner than the right because the:
   A. wall of the left ventricle isn't as thick as the wall of the right ventricle.
   B. left ventricle pushes blood against greater resistance than the right ventricle.
   C. left atrium ejects more blood than the right atrium.

Answer: B. The left ventricle pushes blood against greater resistance than the right ventricle.

2. Signs and symptoms typical of right-sided heart failure include:
   A. crackles and hemoptysis.
   B. dry, hacking cough and suprasternal retractions.
   C. pitting edema of the lower extremities and jugular vein distention.

Answer: C. Right-sided heart failure causes a backflow of blood into the venae cavae. As a result, fluid seeps from capillaries into tissues, causing pitting edema of the lower extremities and jugular vein distention.

3. Signs and symptoms typical of left-sided heart failure include:
   A. crackles and hemoptysis.
   B. dry, hacking cough and suprasternal retractions.
   C. hepatomegaly and renal failure.

Answer: A. Left-sided heart failure causes a backflow of blood into the lungs. As a result, a productive cough may produce hemoptysis (frothy, pink or blood-tinged sputum), crackles and, possibly, signs of pleural effusion.

4. Forward heart failure is caused by:
   A. increased resistance in peripheral blood vessels.
   B. increased blood flow to the left side of the heart.
   C. decreased blood flow to the right side of the heart.

Answer: A. Forward heart failure is caused by poor blood flow to the arteries due to increased peripheral vascular resistance, or afterload.

Scoring

☆☆☆ If you answered all four questions correctly, three cheers! You're our Heart Healthy champ!

☆☆ If you answered three questions correctly, way to go. You could be the next Frank-Starling Scholarship winner!

☆ If you answered two or fewer questions correctly, keep yourself in circulation. You're just a heartbeat away from perfusion proficiency!

2

Preventing heart failure

Key facts

- ◆ Some risk factors for heart failure — such as lifestyle behaviors and diet — can be modified to improve health.
- ◆ To decrease mortality and morbidity from heart failure, care focuses on preventing dyspnea, fatigue, and stress.
- ◆ Compliance with treatment for other cardiac conditions such as hypertension and coronary artery disease can greatly decrease the risk of heart failure.
- ◆ Secondary prevention may include weight monitoring and supplemental oxygen.

Primary prevention

Primary prevention strategies are aimed at modifying risk factors that can lead to heart failure. The best way for a person to prevent heart failure is to maintain a healthy lifestyle.

Stick to it

Emphasize the importance of sticking to the prescribed medication and lifestyle regimens. Avoiding heart failure may become a lifelong need, depending on the cause of the failure, and requires patients to be ever vigilant in their own care.

What you can and can't control

Encourage patients to recognize risk factors that can't be modified — such as the patient's age, sex, and race — and to modify factors that can be changed. Risk factors the patient can control include:
- moderate to high salt intake
- obesity
- lack of exercise
- smoking
- stress. (See *When stress strikes.*)

Salt intake

Because sodium can cause fluid retention, a patient with heart failure needs to reduce his sodium intake. Encourage the patient to read food labels for sodium content (200 mg of salt equals 80 mg of sodium chloride).

Now I get it!

When stress strikes

Hans Selye, who pioneered studies on the effects of stress on the body, outlined a predictable series of stages in the body's reaction to stress. This flowchart depicts those stages.

Physical or psychological stress

↓

Alarm reaction

• Arousal of the central nervous system begins.
• Epinephrine and norepinephrine, along with other hormones, are released and cause an increase in heart rate, myocardial contractility, oxygen intake, and mental activity.

↓

Resistance

• The body responds to the stressor and attempts to return to a balanced state, called homeostasis.
• The individual begins using coping mechanisms.

↓　　　　　　　　　↓

Recovery　　　**Exhaustion**

　　　　　　　　• Unlike the alarm stage, the body can no longer produce hormones.
　　　　　　　　• Organ damage begins.

Those specious spices

The patient should use herbs and spices rather than salt to enhance food flavor. Advise the patient that not all flavor enhancers are sodium-free. For instance, monosodium glutamate and horseradish are notoriously high in sodium.

Explain that the patient can order baked, broiled, or roasted foods at restaurants and should skip gravies, soups, and cheesy dressings. Using un-

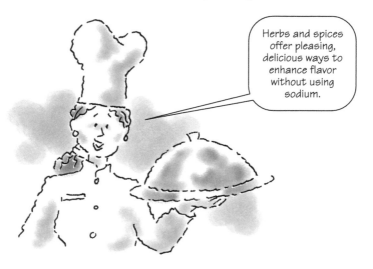

Herbs and spices offer pleasing, delicious ways to enhance flavor without using sodium.

salted meat, broth, soups, butter, and other low-salt foods can also help lower sodium intake.

More salt warnings

Patients with heart failure should avoid salt during cooking and at the table. The patient should also stay away from bottled soft drinks that may contain large amounts of sodium. Low-calorie beverages are particularly high in sodium; manufacturers often substitute sodium saccharin for sugar in these beverages.

Advise patients to consult with their doctor before taking over-the-counter medicines, many of which are high in sodium. For example, Alka-Seltzer, Di-Gel, and Rolaids, commonly used GI medications, are high in sodium. Salt substitutes may be used, pending the doctor's approval, if the patient doesn't have liver or kidney disease.

Obesity

Excess weight causes the heart to work harder. As a result, heart disease is more likely to occur in obese people, even when other risk factors are absent.

Obesity can directly cause a number of cardiac disorders, including hypertension, that can ultimately lead to heart failure. (See *Height and weight table*.) Weight-related definitions you need to know include:

• *normal weight* — 10% above or below recommended weight

• *overweight* — 10% to 20% above recommended weight

• *obese* — 20% or more above recommended weight.

Watching your weight

Weight loss of even 10 to 20 lb (4.5 to 9 kg) can significantly decrease stress placed on the heart. Gradual weight loss, or about 2 to 3 lb (1 to 1.5 kg) per month, is recommended. Explain to your patient that eating a healthy, well-balanced diet holds the key to any successful weight loss.

A dietitian may be helpful in developing a weight-loss diet. Many insurance companies reimburse for the cost of weight-loss assistance. Remind your patient that he should always check with his doctor before starting a weight-loss program.

Height and weight table

Studies suggest that people can carry a bit more weight as they age without added health risk. Because people of the same height may differ in muscle and bone makeup, a range of weights is shown for each height in the table below. The higher weights in each category apply to a man, whose body typically consists of more muscle and bone than that of a woman. Height measurements are given for a person not wearing shoes; weight measurements are given for a person not wearing clothes.

Height	Weight in pounds	
	Ages 19 to 34	Ages 35 and over
5'0"	97 to 128	108 to 138
5'1"	101 to 132	111 to 143
5'2"	104 to 137	115 to 148
5'3"	107 to 141	119 to 152
5'4"	111 to 146	122 to 157
5'5"	114 to 150	126 to 162
5'6"	118 to 155	130 to 167
5'7'	121 to 160	134 to 172
5'8"	125 to 164	138 to 178
5'9"	129 to 169	142 to 183
5'10"	132 to 174	146 to 188
5'11"	136 to 179	151 to 194
6'0"	140 to 184	155 to 199
6'1"	144 to 189	159 to 205
6'2"	148 to 195	164 to 210
6'3"	152 to 200	168 to 216
6'4"	156 to 205	172 to 222
6'5"	160 to 211	177 to 228
6'6"	164 to 216	182 to 234

Keep in mind that rapid weight loss can also cause a strain on the heart muscle.

Lack of exercise

Regular moderate exercise such as walking or bicycling helps the body use its blood supply more efficiently. Your patient should receive 30 minutes of moderate exercise at least 3 days a week. (See *Tips for exercising safely.*) Remind your patient that he should always check with his doctor before starting an exercise program.

Smoking

Smoking narrows blood vessels, creating increased pressure against the heart. If your patient has a long smoking history, he may find it difficult to quit. Suggest the following techniques to help your patient try to quit smoking:

• bupropion (See *All about bupropion,* page 34.)
• hypnosis
• nicotine transdermal systems (Nicoderm)
• nicotine gums or inhalers
• support groups.

Tips for exercising safely

Teach your patients about exercising safely. Offer them these do's and don'ts.

What you should do

• If you've been inactive for a long time, return to exercise gradually.
• Take part in fitness activities, such as walking and swimming, rather than competitive sports such as tennis.
• Warm up and cool down before and after the activity.
• Incorporate flexibility and strengthening exercises into your routine for a well-rounded program.
• Drink plenty of water on warm days.
• Exercise indoors on hot or cold days. Walk in an enclosed mall, for instance, ride a stationary bicycle, or swim in an indoor pool.
• Wait 2 to 3 hours after a heavy meal before exercising. A light snack warrants a 1- to 2-hour wait.
• Avoid hot or cold showers immediately before or after exertion.
• Wear comfortable, lightweight clothes and shoes with adequate support. Dress in layers and remove articles as you warm up.
• Stay alert for symptoms of problems during exercise. If you experience such symptoms, stop exercising and notify your doctor.

What you shouldn't do

• Don't exercise in extreme heat or cold, windy weather, high humidity, or heavy pollution or at high altitudes.
• Don't exercise when you have a fever or don't feel well.
• Don't overexert yourself or become too fatigued. Continuing to exercise when excessively fatigued increases the risk of injury.

All about bupropion

The antidepressant bupropion (Zyban) is commonly used to assist patients in smoking cessation. Treatment usually lasts 7 to 12 weeks. Bupropion may be used in conjunction with nicotine transdermal systems.

Adverse reactions

The most common adverse reactions of bupropion include headache, agitation, and confusion. Other common adverse reactions include insomnia, sedation, tremor, and dry mouth. Arrhythmia and seizures are possible but are less common.

Patient teaching

Advise the patient to take bupropion as scheduled and to take each day's dosage in three divided doses to minimize the risk of seizures. The patient should avoid alcohol while taking this drug because alcohol may contribute to the development of seizures.

Advise the patient to avoid hazardous activities that require alertness and good psychomotor coordination until central nervous system effects of the drug are known. Also advise him to consult his doctor before taking other prescription or over-the-counter medications.

Stress

Physical, mental, and emotional stress increase the workload on the heart. Stress prompts the fight-or-flight response, which increases heart rate and blood pressure. Help your patient understand

and employ a wide variety of coping strategies to reduce stress, including:
- exercising
- attending support groups
- getting sufficient rest
- managing time effectively
- talking to a clergy or family member, a friend, or a nurse, mental health counselor, or other health care provider when angry, depressed, or anxious
- taking an antianxiety agent
- focusing on one thought or on breathing to relax fully. (See *Using relaxation techniques,* pages 36 and 37.)

Secondary prevention

Secondary prevention of heart failure involves treating coronary artery disease (CAD), preventing myocardial infarction (MI), and treating anemia and infections.

Treating CAD

CAD causes loss of oxygen and nutrients to myocardial tissue because of poor coronary blood flow. Atherosclerosis is the most common cause of CAD. In this condition, fatty, fibrous plaques, possibly

(Text continues on page 39.)

Using relaxation techniques

Teach your patients techniques for relaxation to reduce stress and the resulting workload on the heart. This table describes four common relaxation techniques.

Technique	Procedure
Listening to recordings	• Get a tape recorder and cassette (or a CD player and a CD) of your favorite music, comedy routines, or stories. Then sit or lie down in a comfortable position, with your legs and arms uncrossed and relaxed, while you listen through headphones. Close your eyes or stare at a nearby object, and concentrate on the recording. • Imagine yourself floating or drifting with the music, or focus on a pleasant scene or image suggested by the music. When listening to a story, try to imagine every detail described by the storyteller. • Keep time with the music by slapping your thigh, tapping a finger or foot, or nodding your head.
Singing	• Get a tape recorder and cassette (or a CD player and a CD) of your favorite music. Select a song you like. Then mouth the words while you sing it in your mind, or sing the song aloud. • Concentrate all your attention on the song's words and rhythm.

Using relaxation techniques *(continued)*

Technique	Procedure
Using rhythmic breathing	• Stare at an object or a person while you inhale slowly and deeply. Exhale slowly. Continue breathing slowly (but not too deeply) while you count silently, "In...2...3...4. Out...2...3...4." • While performing this exercise, concentrate on how the breathing feels. You may want to close your eyes and imagine air moving slowly in and out of your lungs. Continue to count silently to keep your breathing comfortable and rhythmic. If you begin to feel breathless, breathe more slowly or take deeper breaths.
Using progressive muscle relaxation	• Get comfortable, and close your eyes. Tense the muscles in your forehead and face. Hold this tension for 5 to 10 seconds. • Relax your forehead and face. Hold and enjoy this relaxation for 10 to 15 seconds. • Proceed downward toward your feet, first tensing and relaxing the muscles in your jaw, and then each shoulder, arm, and hand. Do the same for your stomach and buttocks, and then each thigh, lower leg, ankle, and foot. • If you have trouble relaxing some muscles or if the tension causes pain, gently massage that body part until the muscles feel more comfortable. • To complete the exercise, open your eyes, stretch, and relax your entire body. Take a few deep breaths. Don't engage in any activity until you feel fully alert.

Preventing and treating CAD

Treatment for CAD may focus on one of two goals: reducing myocardial oxygen demand or increasing the oxygen supply and alleviating pain. Interventions may be noninvasive or invasive.

Prevention

Overweight patients should limit calories. All patients should limit their intake of salts, fats, and cholesterol and refrain from smoking. Regular exercise is important, though it may need to be done more slowly to alleviate pain. If stress is a known pain trigger, patients should learn stress-reduction techniques.

Other preventive actions include controlling hypertension, reducing serum cholesterol or triglyceride levels with antilipemics, and minimizing platelet aggregation and blood clot formation with aspirin.

Noninvasive treatment

Drug therapy consists mainly of the use of beta blockers or nitrates, such as nitroglycerin or isosorbide dinitrate. Aspirin may also be given to reduce arterial inflammation and help prevent arterial occlusion.

Invasive treatment

Three invasive treatments are commonly used: coronary artery bypass graft (CABG), percutaneous transluminal coronary angioplasty (PTCA), and laser surgery.

CABG. A patient with severely narrowed or blocked arteries may need a CABG to alleviate uncontrollable angina and prevent myocardial infarction (MI). In a CABG, part of the saphenous vein in the leg or the internal mammary artery in the chest are grafted between the aorta and the affected artery beyond the obstruction.

(continued)

Preventing and treating CAD *(continued)*

PTCA. PTCA may be performed during cardiac catheterization to compress fatty deposits and relieve occlusion. In a patient with calcification, this procedure may reduce the extent of the obstruction by fracturing the plaque. PTCA causes fewer complications than surgery, but it does have some risks, including:

- circulatory insufficiency
- MI
- restenosis of the vessels
- retroperitoneal bleeding
- sudden coronary reocclusions
- vasovagal response and arrhythmias
- death (rare).

PTCA is a good alternative to CABG in elderly patients and those who can't tolerate surgery. Patients with occlusion of the left main coronary artery or lesions in extremely tortuous vessels are not candidates for PTCA.

Laser surgery. Laser angioplasty corrects occlusion by vaporizing fatty deposits using a hot-tip laser device. Rotational ablation, or rotational atherectomy, removes plaque using a high-speed, rotating bur covered with diamond crystals.

including calcium deposits, progressively narrow the coronary artery lumens, which reduces the volume of blood that can flow through them. High blood pressure can also lead to CAD and heart failure. (See *Preventing and treating CAD.*)

Preventing MI

Heart failure may be a complication of an MI, so prevention of MI is imperative. Preventive measures include weight control, smoking cessation, exercise, and a reduction of salt intake. Other preventive measures include diet and alcohol modification and awareness of warning signs and symptoms.

Keeping to a low cholesterol diet

Teach the patient how to reduce his risk of MI and heart failure through dietary modifications such as reductions in cholesterol and saturated fat intake. Instruct him to limit his cholesterol intake to under 300 mg/day and his fat intake to less than 30% of total calories. Explain the benefits of adding fiber, fish, and olive oil to the diet. A dietitian's input can be invaluable in helping a person make these and other dietary changes.

Avoiding alcohol

If the patient drinks alcoholic beverages, advise him to limit his daily intake to no more than 1 oz (30 ml) of ethanol (equivalent to 2 oz [60 ml] of 100-proof whiskey, 8 oz [240 ml] of wine or 24 oz

[720 ml] of beer). Explain that alcohol can raise blood pressure and adversely affect the heart. Make sure the patient understands how alcohol interacts with his medications.

Recognizing warning signs and symptoms

Teach your patient how to respond promptly to signs and symptoms of MI. He should notify his doctor if he experiences chest pain, dizziness, excessive shortness of breath, rapid or irregular pulse rate, or prolonged recovery time after exercise or sexual activity.

Treating anemia

In a patient with anemia, cardiac output increases to meet the oxygen demands of body tissues. Routine blood counts for patients with a history of anemia should be performed. If hemoglobin levels drop, consider the infusion of packed red blood cells. If a patient is participating in a bloodless care program, an iron supplement and erythropoietin injections may be used.

Treating infections

Infections increase metabolic demands on the body and thus further burden the heart. All infections should be identified and treated. Instruct the patient to notify his doctor if signs and symptoms of infection appear, such as fatigue, fever, and chills.

Other preventive strategies

Secondary prevention of heart failure also involves strategies to prevent illness and, ultimately, death in patients diagnosed with heart failure. You'll need

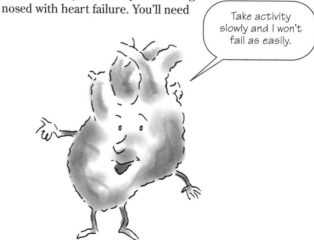

Take activity slowly and I won't fail as easily.

to take several steps to reduce the risk or severity of complications in your patient with heart failure:

• reduce the patient's fatigue by spacing out activities of daily living
• increase activity slowly and gradually
• advise the patient to avoid strenuous exercise.

Romance and candlelight

Advise the patient to reduce his fatigue during sexual activity by waiting 1 to 2 hours after meals before engaging in sex. The patient should also be cautioned to use nonstrenuous positions for intercourse. (See *Resuming sex,* page 44.) A nonstrenuous position involves the at-risk partner lying on his back with pillows propping his head up and his partner on top.

Maintain comfort

Nocturnal dyspnea can be reduced by having the patient sleep on pillows or by elevating the head of the bed. Supplemental oxygen should be used as needed. (See *Types of home oxygen equipment,* pages 45 and 46.) Be sure to teach the

(Text continues on page 47.)

Advice from the experts

Resuming sex

Teach your patient how and when to resume sexual relations after a lengthy illness. Encourage your patient to voice his concerns. Offer the patient these guidelines to help him return to a satisfying sex life:

• Choose a quiet, familiar setting for sex. Strange environments may cause stress. Make sure the room temperature is comfortable. Excessive heat or cold makes your heart work harder.

• Have sex when you're rested and relaxed. A good time is in the morning, after you've had a good night's sleep.

• Don't have sex when you're tired or upset. Avoid having sex after drinking a lot of alcohol. Alcohol expands your heart vessels, which makes your heart work harder. After a large meal, avoid sex for 2 to 3 hours.

• Choose relaxing positions and those that permit unrestricted breathing. Any position that's comfortable for you is okay. Don't be afraid to experiment. At first, you may be more comfortable if your partner assumes the dominant role. You may want to avoid positions that require you to use your arms to support yourself or your partner.

A few precautions

Tell the patient that it's normal for his pulse and breathing rates to rise during sex. They should return to normal within 15 minutes. Advise him to call his doctor at once if he experiences any of these signs or symptoms after sex:

• sweating or palpitations lasting 15 minutes or longer
• breathlessness or increased heart rate lasting 15 minutes or longer
• sleeplessness after sex or extreme fatigue the next day
• chest pain. (The doctor may suggest the use of nitroglycerin prior to sex.)

Running smoothly

Types of home oxygen equipment

To relieve shortness of breath, your patient may need oxygen therapy at home. Oxygen may be supplied using liquid oxygen, pressurized oxygen, or an oxygen concentrator.

• Liquid oxygen is stored at very cold temperatures in insulated containers. When released, the oxygen is warmed up. As the oxygen warms, it turns to gas.

• A stationary liquid oxygen unit typically has a contents indicator that shows the amount of oxygen in the unit, a flow selector that controls flow rate, a humidifier bottle that connects to a humidifier adapter, and a filling connector that attaches to a matching connector on the portable unit.

• An oxygen tank stores oxygen gas under pressure. The tank has a pressure gauge that shows how much oxygen is left, a flow meter that shows the flow rate, and a humidifier bottle.

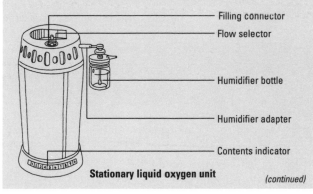

Filling connector
Flow selector
Humidifier bottle
Humidifier adapter
Contents indicator

Stationary liquid oxygen unit

(continued)

Types of home oxygen equipment *(continued)*

• An oxygen concentrator removes nitrogen and other components of room air, and then concentrates the remaining oxygen and stores it.

• When using an oxygen concentrator, check the air inlet filter before operating the unit. If the filter is dirty, wash it with soap and water, rinse it, and pat it dry before replacing it. Push the power switch once to check the alarm buzzer. If the buzzer doesn't sound, use a different oxygen source. If it does sound, push the power switch again to turn it off.

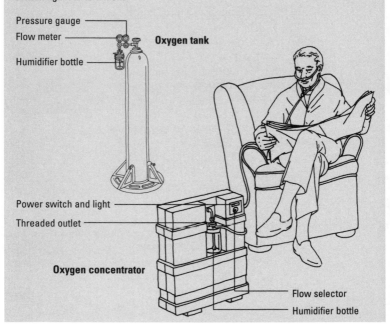

Pressure gauge
Flow meter
Humidifier bottle
Oxygen tank

Power switch and light
Threaded outlet
Oxygen concentrator
Flow selector
Humidifier bottle

patient how to use the oxygen supply equipment at home. (See *Teaching about oxygen supply devices,* page 48.)

Give him the 2-lb warning

Encourage the patient to weigh himself daily at the same time each day on the same scale, wearing the same amount of clothing. Tell him to keep an accurate record of daily weights and to notify his doctor if he notices weight gain. A weight gain of more than 2 lb (1 kg) per day or 3 to 5 lb (1.5 to 2 kg) per week should be reported to the doctor.

OK for U.O.

Monitor urine output while the patient is confined to a health care facility and advise him to monitor it at home as well. Check for decreased urine output, which might indicate that his heart failure has worsened.

And further more...

Make sure the patient knows other reportable signs and symptoms of possible impending heart failure, including anorexia, dyspnea on exertion, persistent

No place like home

Teaching about oxygen supply devices

When teaching about oxygen supply devices, offer these guidelines:
• Check the level of water in the humidifier bottle. If it's below the correct level, refill the bottle with sterile or distilled water or replace it with a new prefilled bottle.
• Attach one end of the oxygen tubing to your breathing device. Attach the other end to the humidifier nipple.
• Set the flow rate using the appropriate method for your device. You may need to turn a dial to the correct number or until a metal ball rises to the correct level on a scale. Or you may need to wait for the gauge needle to reach the correct level.
• After setting the flow rate, put on the breathing device and breathe the oxygen for as long as has been prescribed.

Turning on the flow

• If you're using a liquid oxygen system, turn on the unit by setting the flow rate.
• If you're using an oxygen tank, open the tank before setting the flow rate. To open the tank, turn the valve at the top counterclockwise until the needle on the pressure gauge moves.
• If you're using a concentrator, plug the power cord into a grounded electrical outlet and push the power switch before setting the flow rate. Never increase the flow rate on your own equipment without permission from your doctor.

cough, frequent urination at night, and swelling of ankles, feet, or abdomen. The patient's condition makes him more susceptible to pneumonia and other respiratory infections. Warn him to limit his exposure to crowds and to people with infections. Suggest asking the doctor about the need for pneumonia and influenza vaccinations.

Follow through

Encourage the patient to see his doctor regularly for assessment. Some facilities conduct heart failure clinics, which can help patients incorporate preventive strategies into their daily lives. Regardless of the setting, provide and encourage a calm environment to help reduce stress and allay anxiety.

Quick quiz

1. Flavor enhancers typically high in sodium include:

    A. black pepper.

    B. horseradish.

    C. oregano.

Answer: B. Such flavor enhancers as horseradish and monosodium glutamate are notoriously high in sodium.

2. A patient should report a weight gain of :

    A. 3 lb/day
    B. 2 lb/week
    C. 2 lb/day

Answer: C. A weight gain of more than 2 lb (1 kg) per day or 3 to 5 lb (1.5 to 2 kg) per week should be reported.

3. A patient with heart failure should avoid stress because it can lead to:

    A. central nervous system depression.
    B. increased oxygen demand.
    C. reduced myocardial contractility.

Answer: B. Stress increases heart rate and myocardial oxygen demand.

Scoring

☆☆☆ If you answered all three questions correctly, take a bow. You're the Head Herb on the heart-smart spice rack!

☆☆ If you answered two questions correctly, way to go. Implement some secondary review measures and you'll be hale and hearty in no time.

☆ If you answered fewer than two questions correctly, not to worry. A burst of humidified oxygen should perk you up!

3

Assessing patients with heart failure

Key facts

♦ The most common signs and symptoms of heart failure are dyspnea, edema, and chronic cough.

♦ A cardinal sign of heart failure is an S_3, also known as a gallop.

♦ A full assessment of a patient with heart failure involves taking a health history, conducting a physical examination, and evaluating laboratory results.

Taking a health history

Knowledge of a patient's entire health history is critical for ensuring effective treatment for heart failure. If your patient has acute heart failure, you may not be able to obtain a complete health history because you need to relieve symptoms first. (See *Signs and symptoms of heart failure,* page 52.) When it's appropriate to obtain a health history, ask first about the patient's current complaints and then about health history.

Signs and symptoms of heart failure

Watch for these signs and symptoms of heart failure, divided here according to whether they appear early or late in the disorder.

Early
- Exertional, nocturnal, or paroxysmal dyspnea
- Fatigue
- Hepatomegaly

Late
- Anorexia
- Chest tightness
- Cyanosis
- Dependent edema
- Diaphoresis
- Dullness over lung bases
- Hemoptysis
- Hypotension
- Inspiratory crackles
- Marked hepatomegaly
- Narrow pulse pressure
- Nausea
- Oliguria
- Pallor
- Palpitations
- Pitting ankle edema
- Presence of S_3
- Sacral edema in bedridden patients
- Slowed mental response
- Tachypnea
- Unexplained, steady weight gain

How do you feel now?

In most cases, signs and symptoms of heart failure result from expanding blood volume, congestion of the pulmonary and systemic vascular beds, and excessive sodium and water retention. Patients with heart failure often cite specific complaints, including:

- chest pain
- cough
- fatigue
- dyspnea on exertion, upon lying down, or at night
- swelling of extremities
- weakness.

If your patient is in acute heart failure, relieve his symptoms first. Get a complete health history later.

Left = pulmonary; right = systemic

Heart failure commonly affects both the left and right side of the heart. As a general rule, however, expect to see pulmonary signs and symptoms with left-sided heart failure and systemic signs and symptoms with right-sided heart failure.

Tell me about your (medical) past...

Ask the patient about his medical and family history. Find out what medications he takes, including herbal and other over-the-counter medicines. Ask about previous hospitalizations or treatments for heart failure and about lifestyle behaviors, including smoking and diet.

Also ask about:
• activities of daily living
• sodium intake
• history of anemia, thyroid disease, irregular heart rhythms or palpitations, or recent infection.

...and your family's medical past

Ask whether any relative was diagnosed with heart failure or was suspected of having it. Information about heart failure in family members may help identify underlying causes of the disease and thus select more appropriate treatment options.

Examining a patient with heart failure

Physical examination of a patient with heart failure can yield a great deal of information about the patient's cardiovascular condition and overall physical shape. During the examination, be aware

of landmarks on the chest and the underlying structures. (See *Cardiovascular
landmarks,* pages 56 and 57.)

To assess a patient with heart failure,
use the techniques of inspection, palpa-
tion, percussion, and auscultation. Let's
examine each facet of this examination.

Inspection

First, take a moment to assess the patient's general appearance. Is the patient
alert? Confused? Anxious? Patients experiencing respiratory distress typically appear anxious.

What position?

How is the patient positioned — sitting,
lying, or using pillows? Can the patient
finish a sentence or is he too short of
breath?

The breath that pauses

Deep respirations alternating with short
periods of apnea is the typical respiratory
pattern in patients with heart failure.
(See *Classifying dyspnea,* page 58.) Note if
the patient is showing signs of an abnormal respiratory pattern.

Cardiovascular landmarks

Complete assessment of a patient with heart failure requires an understanding of cardiovascular landmarks. These illustrations show where to find critical landmarks used in a cardiovascular assessment.

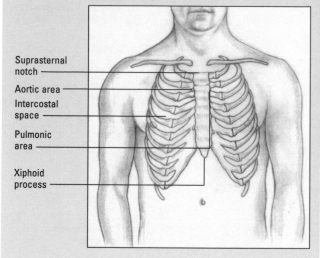

Anterior thorax

Suprasternal notch

Aortic area

Intercostal space

Pulmonic area

Xiphoid process

Cardiovascular landmarks *(continued)*

Lateral thorax

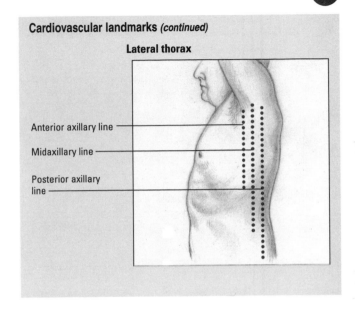

Anterior axillary line

Midaxillary line

Posterior axillary line

Bulging jugulars

You'll also need to inspect the patient for distention of the jugular veins. Here's how:

 Have the patient lie on his back.

 Elevate the head of the bed 30 to 45 degrees.

Classifying dyspnea

Use the New York Heart Classification to classify your patient's dyspnea. This classification system, outlined below, enables you to assess your patient as objectively as possible.

Functional Class I

Normal levels of activity don't promote dyspnea, fatigue, or angina.

Functional Class II

Normal levels of activity promote dyspnea, fatigue, and angina.

Functional Class III

Lower than normal levels of activity promote dyspnea, fatigue, and angina.

Functional Class IV

Dyspnea, fatigue, and angina occur at rest.

Turn the patient's head slightly away from you.

Observe for a pulsation of the jugular vein. Normally, the highest pulsation occurs no more than 1.5″ (4 cm) above the sternal notch. Pulsations that appear higher indicate increased central venous pressure and jugular vein distention.

As you inspect for jugular vein distention, also inspect the skin for pallor or

Peak technique

Assessing patients with dark skin for cyanosis and pallor

To assess dark-skinned patients for cyanosis and pallor, follow these tips:
• Check for pallor of the lips, mucous membranes, and nail beds.
• Check for cyanosis in the conjunctivae, lips, mucous membranes, and nail beds.
• Check for a lackluster appearance to the skin (signifying pallor), with the absence of underlying red tones.
• Look for a yellow hue on brown skin or gray on very black skin. Both findings indicate pallor.

cyanosis. (See *Assessing patients with dark skin for cyanosis and pallor.*)

Palpation

Palpate the lower extremities for swelling or edema. Edema may indicate heart failure, particularly right-sided heart failure. Assigning a grade to the edema provides a baseline to guide future assessments of the patient's condition. (See *Grading edema,* page 60.)

Peak technique

Grading edema

Assigning a grade to a patient's edema allows consistent assessment of the patient's condition. To assess a patient for edema, press your fingertip firmly into the tissue over a bony surface such as the shin. Hold this position for a few seconds. Note the depth of indentation left by your finger.

Then assign a grade to the edema based on this scale:

Grade +1   Slight indentation
Grade +2   Moderate pitting that lasts for a few seconds
Grade +3   Deep indentation that returns slowly to its original contour
Grade +4   An even deeper indentation that returns more slowly to its original contour

Palpable precordium

Next, palpate the precordium. Using the ball of your hand and then your fingertips, palpate the precordium to find the apical impulse. Remember to use a gentle touch so that you don't obscure pulsations. The apical impulse may be difficult to palpate in an obese patient or one with a thick chest wall.

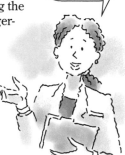

Grading a patient's edema makes it easier to monitor trends,

Can't palpate the apical impulse?

In heart failure, the apical impulse is usually displaced laterally due to an enlarged left ventricle. If the apical impulse proves difficult to palpate with the patient lying on his back, have him lie on his left side or sit or stand upright.

A palpable epigastric pulsation may be an early sign of heart failure.

Percussion

If you suspect cardiomegaly and wish to determine the size of the heart, percussion can help you locate cardiac borders. Begin percussing at the anterior axillary line and percuss toward the sternum along the fifth intercostal space.

Is my apical impulse displaced laterally? It may be because my left ventricle is enlarged.

It's, like, Dullsville, dude

The sound changes from resonance to dullness over the left border of the heart, normally at the midclavicular line. The right border is usually

Estimating liver size

To estimate liver size, use a rule to measure the vertical span between the two marked spots, as shown in this illustration. In an adult, a normal liver span ranges from 2½″ to 4¾″ (6 to 12 cm).

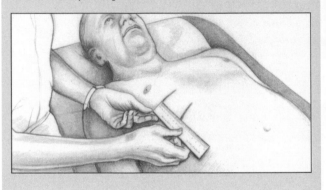

aligned with the sternum and cannot be percussed.

Try a little liver tap

Percussion of the liver can help you estimate its size and determine if the patient has hepatomegaly, a common feature in heart failure. To percuss the liver, ask the patient to take a deep breath and hold it.

Start percussing two finger-breadths below the right nipple along the midclavicular line. You should sense resonance over the lungs. When the resonance changes to dullness, mark the area. The mark indicates the liver's upper border.

Someone tapping, gently tapping, at my liver border

Then, to find the liver's lower border, start percussing about three finger-breadths below the umbilicus. Move upward until the sound changes from tympany to dullness. Mark the spot so you can estimate the size of the liver. (See *Estimating liver size.*)

Percussing the liver can help you gauge liver size and the severity of heart failure.

Auscultation of the heart

Cardiac auscultation requires a methodical approach and lots of practice. Begin by warming the stethoscope with your hands and identifying where you'll auscultate.

Proper position

Have the patient lie supine. If you're right-handed, stand at the patient's right side so you can manipulate the stethoscope with your dominant hand. (See *Positioning the patient for chest auscultation.*)

Zig (listen), zag (listen)

Cardiac auscultation involves auscultating the patient over the cardiac valves and at Erb's point, the third intercostal space at the left sternal border. Use a zigzag pattern to auscultate the patient over the precordium. You can start at the apex and work your way upward or at the base and work downward. Whichever approach you use, be consistent.

Diaphragm one way, bell the other

Use the diaphragm to listen as you go in one direction; use the bell as you come back. Be sure to listen over the entire precordium, not just over the valves.

Lub and Dub — What a pair!

Note the heart rate and rhythm. Always identify the first and second heart sounds, named S_1 and S_2. The *lub* you hear is S_1; the *dub* is S_2.

Adventurous adventitious sounds

Listen for adventitious sounds such as the third heart sound, or S_3, a cardinal

Peak technique

Positioning the patient for chest auscultation

If heart sounds are faint or undetectable, try listening to them with the patient seated and leaning forward or lying on his left side. Repositioning the patient may enhance the sounds or make them seem louder by bringing the heart closer to the surface of the chest.

Forward-leaning position

This position is best for hearing high-pitched sounds related to semilunar valve problems such aortic or pulmonic valve murmurs. To auscultate these sounds, place the diaphragm of the stethoscope over the aortic and pulmonic areas in the right and left second intercostal spaces.

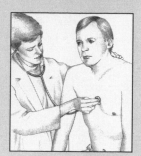

Left-lateral recumbent position

This position is best for hearing low-pitched sounds related to atrioventricular valve problems, such as mitral valve murmurs and extra heart sounds. To auscultate these sounds, place the bell of the stethoscope over the apical area.

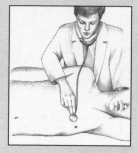

Warning!

The third heart sound

When the mitral and tricuspid valves close in systole, S_1 is produced. When the aortic and pulmonic valves snap shut after ventricular contraction, S_2 is produced.

S_3 is a cardinal sign of heart failure. S_3 immediately follows S_2 in early diastole. S_3 is a low-pitched sound that occurs when the ventricles fill rapidly.

S_3 is often compared to the *y* sound in the word *Kentucky*. This sound is best auscultated at the apex of the heart when the patient is lying on his back.

sign of heart failure. (See *The third heart sound.*)

Auscultation of the lungs

When listening to your patient's breath sounds, auscultate both lung fields — anterior and posterior. (See *Auscultation tips.*) Compare breath sounds on the left to those on the right.

Listen to a full inhalation and full exhalation at each site, using the diaphragm of the stethoscope. Ask the patient to breathe through his mouth; nose breathing alters the pitch of the breathing. Press the stethoscope firmly against the

Peak technique

Auscultation tips

Follow these guidelines as you auscultate your patient for heart sounds:
• Concentrate as you listen to each sound.
• Avoid extraneous sounds by keeping the tubing off the patient's body and other surfaces.
• Use the bell to hear low-pitched sounds and the diaphragm to hear high-pitched sounds.
• Explain that, to ensure a proper assessment, several minutes of listening may be needed to hear all heart sounds. Reassure the patient that extended auscultation doesn't necessarily mean something is wrong.
• Ask your patient to breathe normally and to hold his breath when necessary to enhance sounds that may be difficult to hear.

skin. Also remember not to listen through clothes. The crackle of fabric can sound remarkably like the crackle of fluid in the lungs.

t isn't breakfast cereal

Crackles can be heard when collapsed or fluid-filled alveoli pop open. In a patient with heart failure, crackles occur when the patient stops inhaling. The crackles are usually heard at the bases and in-

Testing for heart failure

Several tests can be used to aid in the diagnosis of heart failure. This list covers the most commonly used of those tests and what results each might show.

• ECG: heart strain, cardiac enlargement, ischemia, atrial enlargement, tachycardia, or extrasystole
• Chest X-ray: increased pulmonary vascular markings, interstitial edema, pleural effusion, or cardiomegaly
• Pulmonary artery pressure: elevated pulmonary artery and capillary wedge pressures, elevated left-ventricular end-diastolic pressure in left-sided heart failure, elevated right atrial pressure or elevated central venous pressure in right-sided heart failure
• Arterial blood gas analysis: decreased Pao_2 (Severe heart failure may cause metabolic acidosis.)

crease in intensity in the upper lung fields.

Laboratory studies

No single test can verify the presence of heart failure. To confirm the condition and gauge its severity, type, and cause, findings from the patient's history, physical examination, and laboratory studies must be weighed. (See *Testing for heart failure*.)

Quick quiz

1. The typical respiratory pattern in patients with heart failure is:

    A. shallow respirations alternating with periods of deep respirations.

    B. deep respirations alternating with periods of shallow respirations.

    C. deep respirations alternating with short periods of apnea.

Answer: C. Deep respirations alternating with short periods of apnea is the typical respiratory pattern in patients with heart failure.

2. When you assess jugular vein distention, place your patient:

    A. in an upright sitting position.

    B. flat on his back in bed.

    C. flat on his back, with the head of the bed elevated 30 to 45 degrees.

Answer: C. Jugular vein distention should be assessed when the patient's head is elevated 30 to 45 degrees.

3. When percussing the precordium to determine heart size, the sound changes from resonance to dullness over the left border of the heart, which is normally located:

    A. over the epigastrium.

    B. at the midaxillary line.

    C. at the midclavicular line.

Answer: C. When percussing the heart, the sound changes from resonance to dullness over the left border of the heart, normally at the midclavicular line.

Scoring

☆☆☆ If you answered all three questions correctly, go to the head of the class. You get an A+ in assessment!

☆☆ If you answered two questions correctly, give yourself a gold star. The signs all point to successful assessment.

☆ If you answered fewer than two questions correctly, consider it history. Assess the situation and try it again.

4

Treating patients with heart failure

Key facts

♦ The human heart can fail from many causes and create a wide array of signs and symptoms. So don't expect to see the same pattern emerge every time.

♦ For most patients, the key elements in treating heart failure are identifying and correcting the underlying causes and managing symptoms.

♦ Surgery may be performed to correct arrhythmia, hypertension, or heart deformities.

♦ Positive inotropic agents increase heart contractility and maximize cardiac function.

♦ Valve surgery, a ventricular assist device, or an intra-aortic balloon pump may be used for a patient with chronic heart failure. If those procedures fail, the patient may undergo heart transplantation.

Drug therapy

Despite the many causes of heart failure, all treatments are aimed at one common goal: to reverse the heart failure, thereby

Battling illness

Guidelines for treating heart failure

The overriding goal of therapy for a patient with heart failure is to improve pump function. This chart highlights key therapeutic goals and the medications and supportive measures used to achieve those goals.

Goal	Therapy
Improve pump performance	• Cardiac glycosides • Other positive inotropic drugs
Reduce cardiac workload	• Vasodilators • Anxiety reduction • Rest • Assisted circulation • Weight reduction
Control salt and water retention	• Diuretics • Low-sodium diet • Mechanical fluid removal
Increase oxygenation	• Oxygen therapy • Rest

improving cardiac function. (See *Guidelines for treating heart failure*.) Drugs play a significant role in reaching that goal.

Gotta luuuuv these drug classes

Drug treatment for heart failure may involve drugs from these classes:
• angiotensin-converting enzyme (ACE) inhibitors
• angiotensin receptor blockers
• beta blockers
• cardiac glycosides
• diuretics
• nitrates.

Positive inotropic drugs

Positive inotropic drugs such as digoxin maximize cardiac performance by increasing ventricular contractility. (See *All about positive inotropic drugs,* page 74.) Digoxin boosts intracellular calcium at the cell membrane, enabling stronger heart contractions. It also produces electrophysiologic changes that decrease conduction speed through the atrioventricular (AV) node.

These effects improve cardiac output. As cardiac output improves, the heart no longer needs to beat faster to compensate for its poor pumping action. As a result, the heart rate slows.

> Ja, I get all pumped up vit digoxin and can contract more forcefully.

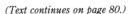

(Text continues on page 80.)

All about positive inotropic drugs

This chart examines indications and dosages, adverse reactions, and special considerations for certain positive inotropics.

Drug	Indications and dosage	Adverse reactions
amrinone Inocor	*For short-term management of heart failure,* give loading bolus of 0.75 mg/ kg I.V. over 2 to 3 minutes. Repeat 30 minutes after initiating therapy. Maintenance dose is 5 to 10 mcg/ kg/minute by infusion.	• Anorexia • Arrhythmia • Hepatotoxicity (rare) • Hypotension • Nausea • Thrombocytopenia • Vomiting
digoxin Lanoxin	*For heart failure, paroxysmal supraventricular tachycardia, atrial fibrillation, and atrial flutter,* the average loading dose for adults, given over 24 hours, is 0.5 to 1 mg I.V. or P.O. given in divided doses.	• Agitation • Anorexia • Arrhythmia (most commonly, conduction disturbances) • Diarrhea • Diplopia • Fatigue • Headache

Special considerations

• Know that amrinone shouldn't be used in patients with severe aortic or pulmonic valvular disease in place of surgical correction of the obstruction or during the acute phase of a myocardial infarction (MI).
• Be aware that amrinone is primarily prescribed for patients who haven't responded to cardiac glycosides, diuretics, or vasodilators.
• Don't administer furosemide and amrinone through the same I.V. line because precipitation occurs.
• Monitor platelet count. If it falls below 150,000/μl, decrease dosage as ordered.
• Know that patients with end-stage cardiac disease may receive home treatment with an amrinone drip while awaiting heart transplantation.
• Be aware that amrinone enhances the inotropic effects of cardiac glycosides.
• Know that when drug is used with disopyramide, excessive hypotension may result.

• Before administering a loading dose of digoxin, obtain baseline data (heart rate and rhythm, blood pressure, and electrolytes) and question the patient about use of cardiac glycosides within the previous 2 to 3 weeks.
• Be aware that the loading dose is divided over the first 24 hours unless the situation indicates otherwise.
• Before giving, take apical-radial pulse for 1 minute. Record and report to the doctor significant changes (sudden increase or decrease in pulse rate, pulse deficit, irregular beats and, particularly, regularization of a previously irregular rhythm). If any occur, check blood pressure and obtain a 12-lead electrocardiogram.

(continued)

All about positive inotropic drugs *(continued)*

Drug	Indications and dosage	Adverse reactions
digoxin *(continued)*	The maintenance dosage is 0.125 to 0.5 mg I.V. or P.O. daily (average is 0.25 mg). Depending on the response, larger dosages may be needed for arrhythmia. In adults over 65 years, the dosage is 0.125 mg P.O. daily as a maintenance dosage. Frail or underweight elderly patients may require only 0.0625 mg daily or 0.125 mg every other day.	• Hallucinations • Malaise • Muscle weakness • Nausea • Paresthesia • Photophobia • Slow or irregular pulse • Visual disturbances (halos around objects) • Vomiting
dobutamine Dobutrex	*To increase cardiac output in short-term treatment of cardiac decompensation caused by depressed contractility, such as during refractory heart failure, or as an adjunct in cardiac surgery,* the usual dosage is 2.5 to 10 mcg/kg/minute by infusion.	• Chest pain • Headache • Hypertension • Hypotension • Increased heart rate • Nausea • Palpitations • Vomiting

Special considerations

• Excessive slowing of the pulse rate (60 beats/minute or less) may be a sign of digitalis toxicity. Withhold the drug and notify the doctor.
• Monitor serum potassium levels. Take corrective action to avoid hypokalemia.
• Encourage the patient to eat potassium-rich foods.
• Know that digoxin interacts with many drugs, including amiloride, amiodarone, diltiazem, nifedipine, diuretics, bicarcillin, antacids, anticholinergics, cholestyramine, colestipol, metoclopramide, and parenteral calcium.

• Use dobutamine cautiously in patients with a history of hypertension. The drug may cause an exaggerated pressor response.
• Don't use with a beta blocker, which may antagonize the effects of dobutamine.
• Be aware that dobutamine may interact with bretylium, general anesthetics, and tricyclic antidepressants.
• Avoid extravasation. Dobutamine may cause an inflammatory response. Change I.V. sites regularly to avoid phlebitis.
• Don't administer this drug through the same I.V. line with other drugs. Dobutamine is incompatible with heparin, hydrocortisone sodium succinate, cefazolin, cefamandole, neutral cephalothin, penicillin, and ethacrynate sodium.
• Monitor serum electrolyte levels, as ordered. The drug may lower serum potassium levels.
• Tell the patient to report adverse reactions promptly, especially dyspnea and drug-induced headache.
• Instruct the patient to report discomfort at the I.V. insertion site.

(continued)

All about positive inotropic drugs *(continued)*

Drug	Indications and dosage	Adverse reactions
dopamine Intropin	*To treat shock and correct hemodynamic imbalances, improve perfusion to vital organs, increase cardiac output, and correct hypotension,* give 1 to 5 mcg/kg/minute by I.V. infusion. The dosage is titrated to the desired hemodynamic or renal response. The infusion rate may be increased by 1 to 4 mcg/kg/minute at 10- to 30-minute intervals.	• Angina • Arrhythmia • Headache • Hypertension • Hypotension • Nausea • Tachycardia • Vasoconstriction • Vomiting
milrinone Primacor	For short-term management of heart failure, give loading dose of 50 mcg/kg I.V. over 10 minutes. Maintenance dose is 0.375 to 0.75 mcg/kg/minute by infusion.	• Headache • Ventricular arrhythmia

Special considerations

• Use dopamine cautiously in patients with occlusive vascular disease, cold injuries, diabetic endarteritis, and arterial embolism; in pregnant patients; in those with sulfite sensitivity; and in those taking monoamine oxidase (MAO) inhibitors.
• Use a central line or large vein to minimize the risk of extravasation. Watch the infusion site carefully for signs of extravasation; if it occurs, stop the infusion immediately and call the doctor. Extravasation may require infiltration with 5 to 10 mg of phentolamine in 10 to 15 ml of normal saline solution.
• Don't mix other drugs in an I.V. container with dopamine. Don't give alkaline drugs through an I.V. line containing dopamine.
• After the administration of dopamine has been stopped, watch closely for a sudden drop in blood pressure. Taper the dosage slowly to evaluate stability of blood pressure, as ordered.
• Be aware that acidosis decreases the effectiveness of dopamine.
• Know that dopamine interacts with alpha blockers, beta blockers, ergot alkaloids, inhalation anesthetics, MAO inhibitors, and phenytoin.
• Instruct the patient to alert a nurse if discomfort occurs at the I.V. site.

• Don't use milrinone in patients with severe aortic or pulmonic valvular disease in place of surgical correction of the obstruction or during the acute phase of an MI.
• Be aware that improved cardiac output may enhance urine output. Expect a dosage reduction in the patient's diuretic therapy as his condition improves.
• Potassium loss may predispose the patient to digitalis toxicity.
• Monitor fluid and electrolyte status, blood pressure, heart rate, and renal function during therapy. An excessive decrease in blood pressure requires discontinuing or slowing the rate of infusion.
• Furosemide infused into an I.V. line containing milrinone forms a precipitate.

Before you give that drug

Key points about two adrenergics

Two inotropic drugs — dopamine and dobutamine — are adrenergics, also called sympathomimetics. For each of these drugs, remember these key points:

• The solution is stable for only 24 hours, so check the label for expiration date and time. Discard the solution if it shows discoloration or a precipitate. (A slightly pink dobutamine solution can be used.)

• Use an infusion pump when administering these drugs. The infusion rate determines the drug's action, so it must be carefully controlled to achieve the desired effect.

• Don't add an alkaline solution, such as sodium bicarbonate, to the solution or infusion line. Alkaline solutions inactivate these drugs.

• Continually monitor the patient's heart rate and rhythm, blood pressure, and urine output.

Backup infusion

If a patient has acute heart failure, the doctor may order I.V. administration of the positive inotropics amrinone or milrinone. Dopamine or dobutamine, both adrenergics, may also be used. (See *Key points about two adrenergics.*) All four drugs improve the heart's pumping ability. Depending on the drug and dose used, they may also dilate peripheral blood vessels. As a result of vasodilation and improved cardiac contractility, pump pressure decreases and overall cardiac workload diminishes.

Diuretics

By increasing urine output, diuretics reduce cardiac preload and make the heart's job easier. These medications, available in

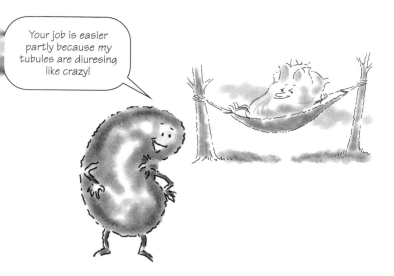

oral and parenteral forms, vary greatly in how they work and which part of the kidney they target. Potency and adverse reactions also differ from drug to drug.

This tubule's got me all convoluted

Diuretics exert various effects depending on which parts of the kidney nephron are involved. For instance, diuretics that target the kidney's proximal tubule generally produce few benefits because activities at other sites may actually reverse the drugs' effects. Potassium-sparing diuretics such as spironolactone and thiazide diuretics such as hydrochlorothiazide act on the proximal and distal convoluted tubules, producing more efficient diuresis.

Get into the loop with loop diuretics

Loop diuretics are the most potent diuretics available. Loop diuretics interfere with chloride and sodium reabsorption at the loop of Henle and improve cardiac function by rapidly decreasing circulating fluid volume.

Examples of loop diuretics include:
- bumetanide
- ethacrynic acid
- furosemide.

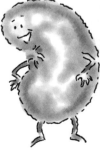

For fast action, go with loop diuretics!

Start slow

Initially, the doctor may prescribe conservative diuretic therapy. Mild diuretics, such as hydrochlorothiazide, may relieve the patient's signs and symptoms and reduce the risk of volume depletion and dehydration. Keep in mind, however, that even mild diuretics can deplete potassium stores.

Too much of a good thing

Although loop diuretics reduce circulating fluid volume rapidly, they also cause more severe adverse reactions than other diuretics. For instance, loop diuretics may cause significant dehydration, thus taking the patient quickly from one extreme — volume overload — to the other — volume depletion.

Potassium-poor

Loop diuretics also typically deplete potassium. Be sure to closely monitor serum potassium and magnesium levels in your patient taking a loop diuretic, and advise the patient to eat high-potassium foods, such as meats, fruits (especially oranges, bananas, apricots, and cantaloupe), vegeta-

> There's nothing like a banana to replace potassium lost through loop diuretic use.

bles (especially potatoes, mushrooms, tomatoes, and carrots), dried fruit, nuts, seeds, and chocolate.

Preload reducers

Preload reducers enhance the effectiveness of positive inotropic drugs and diuretics. Drugs in this class include nitroglycerin and other nitrates.

Preload reducers work by directly relaxing smooth muscles in blood vessel walls and producing generalized dilation. This dilation reduces venous return to the heart, thus decreasing left ventricular end-diastolic pressure (preload). This effect is more pronounced in veins than in arteries.

Afterload reducers

Afterload reducers diminish cardiac workload by decreasing peripheral vascular resistance. Afterload reducers in general work by:
• decreasing myocardial oxygen demand
• increasing renal and cerebral blood flow
• improving cardiac output by facilitating ventricular ejection
• reducing peripheral vascular resistance.

Cuttin' down the afterload

A large number of drugs reduce afterload, including:

- alpha receptor blockers, such as prazosin and doxazosin
- ACE inhibitors, such as lisinopril, enalapril, and captopril
- angiotensin receptor blockers, such as losartan and valsartan
- direct acting vasodilators such as hydralazine
- mixed vasodilators such as nitroprusside.

ACE inhibitors lower blood pressure and reduce arterial resistance without affecting cardiac output. Cool.

Those ace ACE inhibitors

ACE inhibitors, one of the most commonly used classes of afterload reducers, work primarily by interfering with the renin-angiotensin-aldosterone system. These drugs inhibit the enzyme that converts angiotensin I to angiotensin II.

This inhibition slows the release of aldosterone by the adrenal cortex, which, in turn, prevents sodium and water retention. The inhibition of aldosterone release also reduces peripheral arterial resistance and lowers blood pressure without affecting cardiac output or heart rate.

Beta-adrenergic blockers

As the body strains to increase cardiac output, both epinephrine and norepinephrine continuously stimulate the failing heart. The constant flooding of these hormones to the heart reduces the responsiveness of the myocardium to adrenergic stimulation. The solution to this problem is beta-adrenergic blockers, more commonly referred to as "beta blockers."

Beta blockers to the rescue

Beta blockers block the uptake of epinephrine and norepinephrine, thereby increasing myocardial responsiveness.

This increased responsiveness allows the myocardium to react more efficiently to epinephrine (up regulation), thereby enhancing cardiac performance. Carvedilol is the beta blocker of choice for treating heart failure.

Supportive measures

Medical treatment for heart failure also involves several supportive options, including antiembolism stockings and oxygen therapy.

Antiembolism stockings

Bed rest is an essential part of treatment for acute heart failure. However, prolonged bed rest itself may lead to various complications such as venous stasis. Antiembolism stockings are commonly used to prevent venous stasis and thromboembolism.

Pull up your socks!

These stockings apply consistent pressure to superficial blood vessels, thereby giving a boost to blood returning to the heart.

Oxygen therapy

The patient may need supplemental oxygen to improve cardiac function. Oxygen therapy can help the patient keep up with the increased myocardial workload that stems from the heart's attempts to compensate for hypoxemia.

Patients may receive oxygen

> The stockings on your legs will help blood flow back to your heart.

through one of several administration
systems, including:
- nasal cannula
- simple mask
- partial rebreather mask
- nonrebreather mask
- mechanical ventilation.

Surgical options

Surgery for heart failure ranges from
thoracentesis for a patient with chronic
heart failure to implantation of mechanical devices, such as an intra-aortic balloon pump (IABP), to transplantation of
the entire heart.

Thoracentesis

Patients with chronic heart failure may
experience fluid in the pleural cavity as a
result of the buildup of fluid within the
vasculature. If the pleural effusion is
large enough, the fluid may need to be
removed with thoracentesis.

Aspirate that pleura

Thoracentesis involves the aspiration of fluid from the pleural space. Removing this fluid relieves pulmonary compression and respiratory distress.

Intra-aortic balloon pump

If a patient has severe heart failure that can't be controlled with drug therapy, a mechanical device such as the IABP may help maintain cardiac function. (See *How the intra-aortic balloon pump works,* page 90.) The IABP, the most commonly used

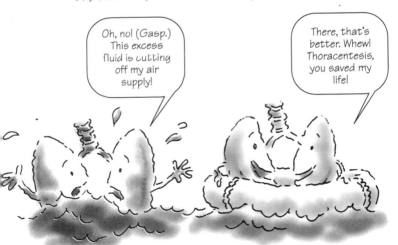

How the intra-aortic balloon pump works

Made of polyurethane, the intra-aortic balloon is attached to an external pump console by a large-lumen catheter. The illustrations here show the direction of blood flow when the pump inflates and deflates the balloon.

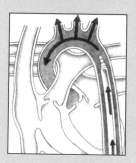

Inflation

The balloon inflates as the aortic valve closes and diastole begins. Balloon inflation increases aortic pressure and improves coronary artery flow.

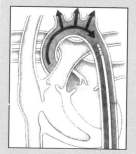

Deflation

The balloon deflates before ventricular ejection, when the aortic valve opens. This permits ejection of blood from the left ventricle against a lower resistance. As a result, aortic end-diastolic pressure and ventricular resistance decrease and cardiac output increases.

device for heart failure, can help sustain a patient's life until the underlying defect can be surgically corrected.

Inserting an IABP

An IABP is typically inserted in the operating room or cardiac catheterization lab. The doctor inserts an intra-aortic balloon percutaneously through the femoral artery and threads it into the descending aorta, slightly beyond the origin of the left subclavian artery.

IABP downside

An IABP can't be used for everyone, nor is it without danger. IABP is contraindicated in patients with aortic aneurysm or other forms of severe aortic disease. In addition, an IABP can cause numerous complications, including:

• arterial embolism
• arterial occlusion and possible loss of limb
• bleeding
• extension or rupture of an aortic aneurysm
• perforation of an artery.

> Yo! Pump me up! A balloon pump can keep me going until I have surgery.

Ventricular assist device

The ventricular assist device (VAD) is a temporary life-sustaining treatment for a failing heart. It diverts systemic blood flow from a diseased ventricle into a centrifugal pump. This diversion temporarily reduces ventricular workload, allows the myocardium to rest, and improves contractility. (See *VADs help failing hearts.*)

Inserting a VAD

A VAD is inserted in an operating room under general anesthesia. The patient is placed on cardiopulmonary bypass, and a midline incision is made into the heart to insert the device. Cannulation sites depend on the type of ventricular support required (right ventricle, left ventricle, or both) and the type of device selected. Heparin is administered to reduce the risk of clotting within the device.

Monitor vital signs and cardiac parameters frequently. If ventricular function fails to improve within 4 days, the patient may need a heart transplant.

VAD downside

Even with vigilant and competent care, complications can arise from the place-

VADs help failing hearts

The ventricular assist device (VAD) functions somewhat like a temporary artificial heart. The VAD, implanted in the patient's chest cavity, assists the workings of one or both ventricles.

The device receives power from a portable battery pack. It can also operate for up to 1 hour at a time using an implanted, rechargeable battery pack. This illustration shows the various components of a VAD.

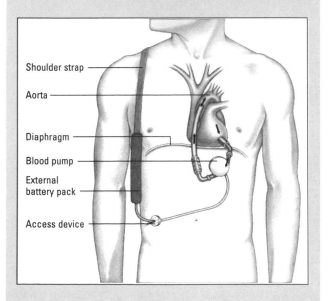

Shoulder strap

Aorta

Diaphragm

Blood pump

External battery pack

Access device

ment of a VAD. These complications include:

- cerebrovascular accident (CVA)
- hemolysis
- pulmonary embolism
- thrombus formation.

Valve replacement

In some cases, the underlying cause of heart failure relates to a problem with a valve — typically the aortic valve or mitral valve. Those patients may require a valve replacement or at least, in the case of the mitral valve, a valve repair.

Natural or artificial?

Surgeons can select either a mechanical or biological valve to replace a diseased or damaged valve. All patients receiving a valve replacement are placed on cardiopulmonary bypass during replacement.

Valve replacement downside

Complications of valve replacement include:
- bacterial endocarditis

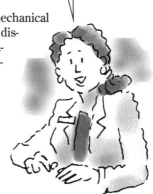

During a valve replacement, the patient will be placed on cardiopulmonary bypass.

- bleeding from long-term anticoagulation therapy
- thrombus formation leading to a CVA
- valve dysfunction or failure.

Heart transplantation

For patients with irreversible heart disease, heart transplantation may be the only viable option. Rigid selection criteria ensure that only those patients with optimal chances of survival are chosen for this procedure.

Patients selected for a heart transplant remain on standard therapy while awaiting a transplant. Other surgical treatments currently under study include the Dor procedure and the Batista surgery. (See *Two new treatment possibilities,* page 96.)

Hurry up and wait

After being accepted for a transplant, the patient is placed on a United Network of Organ Sharing waiting list. The time period before a donor becomes available depends on the patient's blood type and tissue compatibility status.

Two new treatment possibilities

Although still under study, two unusual surgeries to alleviate heart failure have been developed and used successfully in recent years.

Dor procedure

The *endoventricular circular patch plasty,* or the *Dor procedure* (after its developer, Dr. Vincent Dor), involves opening the left ventricle to remove scar tissue and then sewing a patch into the cavity created by removal of the scar tissue. The patch, made of artificial or human tissue, is placed so that it connects areas of strong, properly functioning muscle and excludes areas of scar tissue that interfere with the ventricle's ability to pump blood.

Over time, the patch reshapes the ventricle and improves its function. The procedure is useful for some patients with end-stage heart disease who would benefit from a heart transplant but for whom a donor can't be found in time.

Batista surgery

The Batista surgery is an experimental operation that improves the pumping action of a failing heart by removing a large portion of the left ventricle. This removal improves cardiac contractility. The procedure is used as an alternative to heart transplant in patients with end-stage heart failure.

Now that the transplant is done...

Following a heart transplant, the patient generally remains in the hospital for about 2 weeks. This allows time to fully monitor the patient's heart function and establish stability in the patient's immunosuppressive therapy.

Quick quiz

1. Positive inotropic drugs work primarily by:
    A. dilating blood vessels.
    B. promoting volume reduction.
    C. increasing the force of contraction.

Answer: C. Positive inotropic drugs, such as digoxin and dopamine, increase the force of contraction.

2. Bumetanide and furosemide are diuretics that work directly on the kidney nephrons at the:
    A. glomerulus.
    B. loop of Henle.
    C. proximal tubule.

Answer: B. Bumetanide and furosemide are examples of loop diuretics, which interfere with chloride and sodium reabsorption at the loop of Henle. Furosemide also inhibits sodium and chloride reabsorption in the proximal and distal tubules. Bumetanide acts only on the loop of Henle.

3. Deflation of an IABP occurs during:
A.   early diastole.
B.   early systole.
C.   late systole.

Answer: B. Deflation occurs at the onset of systole and lowers aortic pressure and ventricular resistance. Inflation occurs during diastole and increases aortic pressure and improves blood flow through the coronary artery.

Scoring

☆☆☆   If you answered all three questions correctly, awesome! You've earned a trip to the Inotropical Island Resort at Amrinone Bay.

☆☆   If you answered two questions correctly, groovy, baby. You're heading for the beautiful Southern resort, Tara Transplantation!

☆   If you answered fewer than two questions correctly, ease up. We're putting your name down for a free trip to the Violet Arboretum Display, also known as the VAD. Enjoy!

5

Heart failure complications

Key facts
♦ The three major complications of heart failure are arrhythmia, pulmonary edema, and cardiogenic shock.
♦ Complications of heart failure can occur anytime.
♦ Medications and mechanical ventilatory assistance may be used to treat complications.

Major complications of heart failure

Arrhythmia, pulmonary edema, and cardiogenic shock commonly complicate heart failure. These complications can occur soon after diagnosis or late in patients with chronic heart failure. Assume that regardless of when a patient with heart failure comes under your care, complications could still arise.

Beware! Complications can occur anytime.

Arrhythmia

Abnormal automaticity or changes in electrical conduction within the ventricles as a result of heart failure commonly result in arrhythmia. (See *Recognizing arrhythmias in heart failure.*) The three most common arrhythmias seen in patients with heart failure are:

- atrial fibrillation
- atrial flutter
- ventricular tachycardia.

What's behind the arrhythmia

Atrial fibrillation and atrial flutter may result from enlargement of the atria caused by volume and pressure overload. Ventricular tachycardia results from left ventricular dysfunction, myocardial necrosis, or the development of abnormal conduction pathways in the ventricles.

Treating the arrhythmia

Treatment of arrhythmia focuses on returning pacemaker function to the sinoatrial (SA) node, reestablishing a normal ventricular rate, atrioventricular (AV) synchrony,

I'm all jittery and out of sync from electrical conduction changes. Watch out for arrhythmia!

Don't skip this strip

Recognizing arrhythmias in heart failure

Several arrhythmias are common in patients with heart failure. This chart outlines key features of and treatments for those arrhythmias.

Atrial fibrillation

In atrial fibrillation, the atrial rhythm is grossly irregular and usually indiscernible. You'll see an irregularly irregular ventricular rate, a hallmark sign of this arrhythmia.

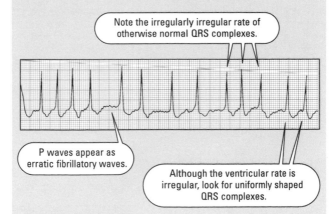

Note the irregularly irregular rate of otherwise normal QRS complexes.

P waves appear as erratic fibrillatory waves.

Although the ventricular rate is irregular, look for uniformly shaped QRS complexes.

(continued)

Recognizing arrhythmias in heart failure *(continued)*

Atrial flutter

In atrial flutter, the atrial rhythm is regular and faster than the ventricular rate, which varies depending on the degree of atrioventricular block. The typical atrial rate is 250 to 400 beats/minute; ventricular, 60 to 100 beats/minute.

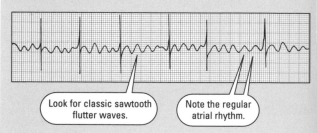

Look for classic sawtooth flutter waves.

Note the regular atrial rhythm.

Ventricular tachycardia

In ventricular tachycardia, a life-threatening arrhythmia, you'll see a ventricular rate of 140 to 220 beats/minute. The rhythm may be regular or slightly irregular.

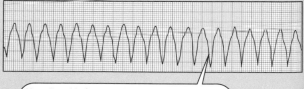

Note the wide (greater than 0.12 second), bizarre QRS complexes. You usually won't see P waves.

and maintaining normal sinus rhythm. Regardless of the arrhythmia, make sure you take the following actions:

• Monitor heart rate and rhythm in every patient with heart failure.

• Obtain a 12-lead ECG to evaluate and document the arrhythmia.

• For a symptomatic patient, start cardiac monitoring and insert an I.V. line using a large-bore catheter (unless one is already in place) to administer emergency drugs.

• Tell the patient to report light-headedness, dizziness, dyspnea, chest pain, altered mental status, or syncope. These signs and symptoms may indicate inadequate cerebral or myocardial perfusion resulting from life-threatening arrhythmia. Also tell the patient to report palpitations, diaphoresis, mild weakness, fear, anxiety, and panic, any of which may be associated with less dangerous arrhythmias.

• Administer drugs as ordered and prepare for corrective procedures such as cardioversion. (See *Treating arrhythmia in heart failure,* page 104.)

• If a patient is unstable and has serious signs and symptoms or a life-threatening arrhythmia, rapidly assess the patient's

Treating arrhythmia in heart failure

This chart examines some of the most common treatment options for two major arrhythmias that occur with heart failure.

Atrial flutter or fibrillation

• If your patient is stable and the ventricular rate is 150 beats/minute or below, prepare to administer drug therapy according to facility protocol. Note that if digoxin or a similar antiarrhythmic caused the arrhythmia, it shouldn't be used for treatment.

• If the patient is stable but has a ventricular rate of more than 150 beats/minute, notify the doctor and follow advanced cardiac life support (ACLS) protocols for tachycardia. If drug therapy is ineffective, the guidelines call for synchronized cardioversion.

• If the patient is stable, but the arrhythmia has persisted, expect to administer anticoagulants to prevent emboli. An embolus may form as a result of loosening of a thrombus adherent to the atrial wall.

• If the patient is unstable, notify the doctor, help determine the cause of the arrhythmia, and monitor the ventricular rate. Administer antiarrhythmic drugs as ordered. If the ventricular rate reaches 150 beats/minute, initiate ACLS protocols for tachycardia.

Ventricular fibrillation

• If the patient is stable, expect to administer lidocaine hydrochloride. Monitor serum electrolyte levels, especially the potassium level.

• If the patient is unstable and is experiencing serious signs and symptoms, prepare for immediate cardioversion, followed by the administration of antiarrhythmic drugs.

• If the patient is pulseless, initiate cardiopulmonary resuscitation. Follow ACLS protocols for defibrillation, endotracheal intubation, and the administration of emergency drugs, including epinephrine, lidocaine, bretylium, magnesium sulfate, and procainamide.

respirations, pulse, and level of consciousness and prepare for defibrillation or cardioversion, according to your facility's protocol. Initiate cardiopulmonary resuscitation, if indicated.

• If your patient's arrhythmia isn't life-threatening and his condition is stable, you may have more time to investigate possible causes of the arrhythmia.

• If the patient has a pulse, notify the primary health care provide and continue to monitor his condition. Never rely on the patient's heart rate alone to determine his hemodynamic stability. Instead, interpret his pulse and ECG findings in light of his appearance.

Pulmonary edema

When left-sided heart failure worsens, pulmonary edema generally follows. Pulmonary edema involves extremely high pressure within pulmonary vessels. (See *Picturing pulmonary edema,* page 106.) This excessive pressure may propel fluid from the vascular space into lung interstitium.

Picturing pulmonary edema

The left ventricle's diminished function causes blood to pool in the left ventricle and atrium, eventually backing up into the pulmonary veins and capillaries, as shown in this illustration. Rising capillary hydrostatic pressure pushes fluid into the interstitial spaces and alveoli, resulting in pulmonary edema.

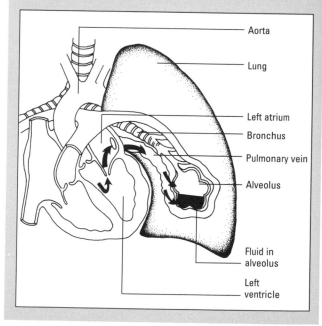

What to look for

Assessing patients for pulmonary edema

The hypoxia and decreased cardiac output of pulmonary edema may make the patient restless, pale or ashen, cool, and sweaty. His vital signs will depend directly on the degree of cardiac compromise, with a more serious condition leading to increasingly worse vital signs.

Other signs and symptoms include:
- air hunger
- crackles or wheezes
- extreme apprehension
- inability to lie flat
- labored breathing
- suffocation sensation
- tachypnea.

Categorizing the condition

How far the resulting pulmonary congestion advances depends on the heart's workload and its ventricular function. (See *Assessing patients for pulmonary edema*.) The extent of pulmonary edema is best described by stages I, II, and III.

In stage I pulmonary edema, the chest's lymphatic system drains fluid away from interstitial spaces. Signs and symptoms may occur with exertion, and pathologic changes may be seen on a chest X-ray.

In stage II, interstitial fluid accumulates faster than the lymphatic system can drain it. As a result, edema develops in the bronchioles, venules, and arteries. Dyspnea, orthopnea, and paroxysmal nocturnal dyspnea occur. Look also for tachypnea, cough, apprehension, and fine crackles over both bases on auscultation.

In stage III, the most advanced stage, alveolar edema develops from excessive pulmonary pressure and rapid fluid transudation from vascular and interstitial spaces into alveoli. (See *Emergency intervention for pulmonary edema.*) This condition creates an extreme impairment in oxygen exchange. Look for severe dyspnea, dangerously low blood oxygen levels, and moist crackles throughout the lung fields on auscultation.

Memory jogger

To help you remember the three primary complications of heart failure, put on your thinking CAP.

Cardiogenic shock

Arrhythmia

Pulmonary edema

Battling illness

Emergency intervention for pulmonary edema

If your patient's heart failure deteriorates to pulmonary edema, intervene quickly and efficiently. Here's how.

Do this first...

• Call for help. Notify the doctor at once, and gather emergency equipment.
• Assess and ensure airway patency and oxygenation. Maintain proper airway position. Encourage coughing, if the cough is productive. Suction only if absolutely necessary, to avoid further decreasing oxygen levels. Administer oxygen by mask or nasal cannula. Prepare intermittent positive-pressure breathing treatment, and draw a blood sample for arterial blood gas levels, as ordered.
• Position the patient to decrease venous return. If possible, place him in high Fowler's position, letting his legs dangle to further decrease venous return. Monitor his blood pressure closely.
• Start an I.V. line with a large bore catheter. Choose an insertion site unaffected by position changes.

...And then this

• Assess vital signs routinely. Check his vital signs frequently until his condition stabilizes.
• Monitor heart rate and rhythm. Attach a cardiac monitor, and observe closely for arrhythmia.
• Administer drugs, as ordered. Prepare to give I.V. furosemide, morphine, digoxin, or other drugs, as ordered.
• Calculate strict fluid intake and output. Prepare to insert an indwelling urinary catheter to monitor output. Restrict fluids.
• Provide emotional support. Reassure the patient and his family.

Now I get it!

Cycle of cardiac deterioration

Even a slight reduction in arterial pressure can trigger a cycle of cardiac deterioration from diminished coronary blood flow. This illustration demonstrates the dangerous cycle.

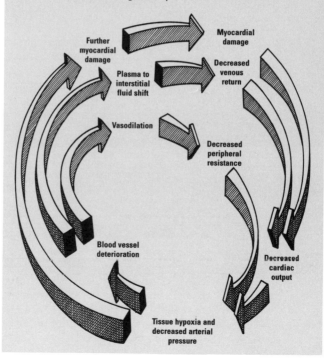

Perils of pulmonary edema

Without intervention, the patient's condition can deteriorate quickly and become perilous. Pulmonary edema can rapidly lead to marked hypotension, cardiogenic shock, and ultimately death. Treatment is aimed at reducing fluid volume and improving oxygenation.

Cardiogenic shock

Cardiogenic shock stems from severe circulatory failure as a result of impaired pumping ability. (See *Cycle of cardiac deterioration.*) Signs and symptoms include:
- cold, clammy skin
- confusion
- cyanosis
- diaphoresis
- diminished urine output
- rapid, thready pulse
- restlessness.

Turn to dopamine, positive inotropics, and vasopressors when complications arise.

Treating complications

Treatment for a patient with complications of heart failure is aimed at increasing cardiac output, improving myocardial perfusion, and decreasing cardiac workload. Treatment may involve drugs or mechanical assist devices.

Drug therapy

Dopamine, a vasopressor, can be used to increase cardiac output, blood pressure, and renal blood flow. Positive inotropic drugs, such as dobutamine and amrinone, increase myocardial contractility. When a more potent vasopressor is necessary, norepinephrine may be used.

Nitroprusside to the rescue!

Nitroprusside, a potent vasodilator, may be used to improve cardiac output. This drug decreases peripheral vascular resistance (afterload) and reduces left ventricular end-diastolic pressure (preload). However, the patient's blood pressure must be adequate before nitroprusside administration and should be monitored closely after administration.

Mechanical assistance

When cardiogenic shock stems from a mechanical defect, an intra-aortic balloon pump (IABP) can provide effective temporary assistance until surgery cor-

> Sometimes I need a little high-tech help. Enter IABP.

rects the defect. If the shock results from extensive myocardial damage, however, other therapies may prove more suitable. Weaning the patient off an IABP when the heart has experienced extensive damage may prove difficult. In those cases, the existing muscle may not be able to sustain sufficient cardiac output without the pump.

Quick quiz

1. One of the most common complications of heart failure is:

    A. ventricular fibrillation.

    B. ventricular standstill.

    C. ventricular tachycardia.

Answer: C. Ventricular tachycardia commonly occurs because of left ventricular dysfunction with myocardial necrosis and development of the reentry pathways.

2. Signs and symptoms of cardiogenic shock are caused by:

    A. an increased cardiac output.

    B. a decreased cardiac output.

    C. hypoxic tissues.

Answer: B. Signs and symptoms that occur with cardiogenic shock result from decreased cardiac output.

3. Cardiogenic shock may develop from:
   A. increased function of the ventricle.
   B. decreased function of the ventricle.
   C. increased cardiac output.

Answer: B. Cardiogenic shock results from a marked decrease in functional ventricular muscle tissue.

Scoring

☆☆☆ If you answered all three questions correctly, that is, like, soooo cool. We're giving you this totally awesome Amazing Arrhythmia award for, like, you know, being so *there,* you know?

☆☆ If you answered two questions correctly, ooooh, dude. Too cool. Here's a ticket to the newest nightclub in town, Pulmonary Edema Stage 54. Have a blast!

☆ If you answered fewer than two questions correctly, whoa! How about a free copy of Interstitial Fluid Shift, a most *out there* movie starring Pree Lode and Phineas P. Crackles? Excellent!

6

Teaching patients with heart failure

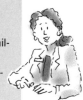

Key facts
♦ Be aware of cultural differences that may affect your patient teaching about heart failure.
♦ Teaching about diet, weight loss, and medications can help improve compliance.
♦ Activity should be limited only in early stages of heart failure. In later stages, patients should remain as active as possible.

Teaching strategies

Help your patient understand how he can live a long, healthy life despite having heart failure. Teach him about:
• the reason his diet will need to change and the way he will need to change it
• the importance of exercise and recommended activity
• drugs for heart failure, their function, and their adverse effects
• symptoms he should report to the doctor.

> ### Causes of heart failure
> - Diabetes
> - Myocardial infarction
> - Obesity
> - Uncontrolled hypertension

Assess learning needs

Before initiating a teaching program about heart failure causes, risk factors, complications, and treatment, assess your patient's learning needs. Determine whether language difficulties or cultural differences exist as well as how ready the patient is to learn. Then plan your teaching carefully.

Speaking the language

Make sure your patient understands English, and if not, make sure instructions are translated into the person's native language or give instructions to a family member who speaks English. Photos or illustrations can prove valuable for patients who can't speak English fluently.

> ### Heart failure risk factors
> - Alcohol abuse
> - Cardiomyopathy
> - Family history of heart failure
> - High cholesterol levels
> - Obesity
> - Smoking

Understand cultural influences

Be aware of cultural differences that might affect your patient's comprehension. When possible and appropriate, have someone from the patient's home community with you during teaching sessions.

Ready...or not?

Gauging learner readiness is critical to ensuring that your teaching is effective. Is your patient anxious about his diagnosis or condition? Is he involved in difficult family issues or other emotionally charged situations? Does he refuse to believe the diagnosis or its implications?

Anxiety, emotional upset, denial, and numerous other conditions tend to make learning less effective. Knowing your patient's readiness to learn can help you prepare your teaching plan and initiate teaching when the patient is ready for it.

Make a teaching plan

Making a teaching plan can help organize instruction and promote learning and retention. Here are some tips for educating any patient.

• Break the instructions into small, goal-oriented sessions.

• Keep learning goals achievable.

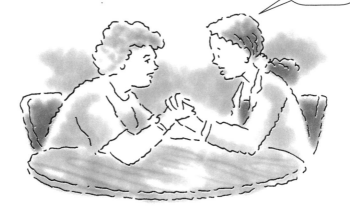

I can see you have a great deal on your mind. Let's talk about diet changes later.

• Make sure the patient or family member can demonstrate what they've been taught.
• Plan your teaching for times when family members are present.
• Talk about the patient's fears and his family's feelings about the disease.
• Choose teaching times when the patient is well rested and comfortable.

Joy of repetition

Most people need facts repeated three or more times before they remember them accurately. Always repeat key points and, for procedures, ask the patient to return-demonstrate the procedure at least once.

Very varied teaching styles

Use different methods of teaching, such as verbal explanation, illustrations on paper, videotape, and actual demonstrations. Using a variety of teaching techniques helps you more effectively meet individual learning needs.

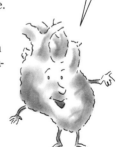

Déja vu all over again can be a good thing.

Teaching about diet changes

A patient with heart failure needs to understand the importance of changing his eating habits, particularly limiting salt and fat intake, cutting down on caffeine, and monitoring his fluid intake.

Limit salt intake

Tell the patient the importance of keeping his sodium level down. Point out that a low-sodium diet (2 to 3 g/day) increases urine output and helps prevent fluid accumulation. (See *Cutting down on salt.*)

Limit fat intake

Because fat can contribute to coronary artery disease, a primary cause of heart failure, tell the patient to:
- eat less red meat and processed meat
- eliminate lard from the diet
- limit intake of dairy products, especially whole milk
- limit intake of saturated tropical oils, such as coconut, palm, and palm kernel oil. Olive oil may be used instead.

Other fat-limiting steps include:
- trimming visible fat from red meat
- removing the skin from poultry before cooking

Teaching about diet changes

Cutting down on salt

Advise the patient to reduce salt intake to a teaspoon or less a day.
Offer these tips:

- Use less table salt.
- If indicated, substitute a salt replacement such as NoSalt in cooking and at the table.
- Read the label on all foods, and avoid those that contain high
amounts of sodium.
- Avoid prepared foods, especially frozen dinners, canned vegetables, canned soups, catsup, tomato sauce, and peanut butter. These
foods are high in sodium.
- Follow the doctor's instructions about your particular level of sodium restriction.

- substituting fish and margarine for meat
and butter
- broiling, microwaving, grilling, or roast-
ing meat on a rack, and avoiding deep-
frying
- ordering restaurant foods cooked in un-
saturated vegetable oils only
- eating no more than three egg yolks in
1 week, including yolks in prepared foods.

What? More limits?

Tell the patient to taper caffeine and alcohol use as well. Caffeine may overstimu-

late the heart and nerves, leading to arrhythmia, and raise the blood pressure. The patient should also limit alcohol intake because alcohol decreases the heart's ability to contract.

Fruits, veggies, and fishies for potassium

Patients taking potassium-depleting diuretics or certain other drugs may need to increase their potassium intake. These foods are excellent sources of potassium:

- avocados
- bananas
- cantaloupes
- carrots
- dates
- green leafy vegetables
- potatoes
- salmon.

Following up on fluid intake

The patient need not restrict his fluid intake unless instructed by his doctor. To determine if fluid restrictions are necessary, tell the patient to:

- monitor his fluid intake and approximate output
- weigh himself daily

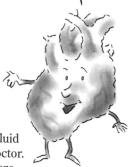

Replacing potassium lost to potassium-depleting diuretics can help prevent arrhythmia — a real plus for me!

• log each measurement in a diary
• report a weight gain of 3 lb (1.5 kg) or more in 1 week to his doctor.

Dieting for better health

An overweight patient with heart failure should be encouraged to lose weight. Weight loss lowers blood pressure and eases breathing difficulties. Encourage your patient to limit intake of fatty foods

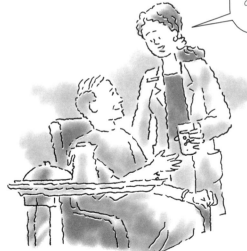

and foods high in calories. In addition, advise your patient to exercise regularly. Provide information about approved weight loss programs in his area.

Teaching about drug therapy

Because drug therapy is key in the treatment of heart failure, your patient needs to understand each drug he has been prescribed. For each drug, teach him:
- how the drug works
- how and when to take the drug
- what the possible adverse reactions are and when to alert the doctor
- how to avoid adverse reactions, particularly dizziness and hypotension
- what drugs may interact with the prescribed drugs
- why it's important to comply with the prescribed therapy.

In addition, provide the patient with a wallet-size card listing the drugs he's taking and emergency phone numbers.

Heart failure sites on the Internet

Check out these Internet sites for more information about heart failure.

American Heart Association

www.americanheart.org

This site defines heart failure and provides a short description of how it's diagnosed and treated. It also provides links to other sites. You might check this site to get started on your research.

Heart Point

www.heartpoint.com

This comprehensive site is organized using a series of questions about heart failure. Readers can go directly to the area that interests them or read the entire site to obtain a detailed review of heart failure. The site contains definitions of heart failure and related terms, causes of heart failure, symptoms, tests to assess heart failure, information on prognosis, medication information, and other related facts. You might advise your patient with heart failure to start at this site when looking for general information about his condition.

The Johns Hopkins University

www.med.jhu.edu/heart

This site, from the renowned Johns Hopkins University, provides definitions of heart failure, causes, patient evaluation data, information about new treatments and procedures, heart transplant options, referral informatino, pertinent photographs, a review of heart failure studies, and related links. The liberal use of flowcharts, tables, and other graphics makes this an excellent site for health care professionals looking for information about heart failure, though patients might also find the site useful.

(continued)

Heart failure sites on the Internet *(continued)*

Mayo Clinic

www.mayohealth.org

This site provides the full text of articles printed in the esteemed "Mayo Clinic Health Letter" and includes definitions of heart failure, symptoms, information about the use of various heart failure drugs, and links to other sites. One of the pages *(www.mayohealth.org/mayo/common/htm/heartpg.htm/)* offers an excellent overview of the heart. Check this site to review information about the heart or to research articles in the "Mayo Clinic Health Letter."

Merck

www.merck.com

This site, by the pharmaceutical firm Merck, Inc., provides a general overview of heart failure for patients. Easy to read and understand, the site addresses what heart failure feels like, what doctors look for, what treatment options are availble, and the importance of taking drugs as directed. Refer your patient to this site for clear, comprehensive information about heart failure.

National Heart, Lung, and Blood Institute

www.nhlbi.nih.gov/nhlbi/cardio

This government site provides a thorough review of the incidence, prevalence, and prognosis for heart failure, with content directed toward health care professionals more than patients. Check this site for wide-ranging statistics about heart failure and graphics related to the condition.

Sharp Foundation for Cardiovascular Research and Education and the San Diego Cardiac Center

www.heartfailure.org

This site contains simple explanations of complex concepts involved in heart failure. It explains how the heart works, what heart failure is, and how to better live with heart failure. It also answers frequently asked questions and provides links to related sites. Advise your patient to point his Web browser to this comprehensive site for basic information about his disease.

Heart failure sites on the Internet *(continued)*

Texas Heart Institute

www.sleh.com

This interesting site offers stories of patients with heart failure and explains how treatment for the condition can help. It also reviews new treatments for heart failure. Check this site for first-person information about living with heart failure.

Dabbling with digoxin

Digoxin, commonly used to treat heart failure, strengthens and regulates heart contractions and causes the heart rate to slow. Teach the patient taking digoxin to measure his pulse rate daily. If it falls below 60 beats/minute, he should call his doctor immediately.

Tell the patient also to report these signs and symptoms of toxicity:
- confusion
- dizziness
- drowsiness
- fatigue
- flulike symptoms (elderly patients)
- headache
- loss of appetite

Hey, hey, hey! My rate's dropping below 60!

- malaise
- nausea or vomiting
- slow or irregular pulse
- visual disturbances, such as blurred vision or yellowish-green halos around objects.

When to take digoxin

If the patient is also taking cholestyramine, a lipid-lowering drug, tell him to take it 2 to 3 hours after taking digoxin. Taken concurrently, cholestyramine can decrease digoxin bioavailability or circulating blood levels of digoxin.

Also tell the patient to take digoxin at least 1 hour before taking an antacid or eating high-bran foods, either of which can reduce the bioavailability of digoxin.

Teaching about tests

Help your patient understand tests used to diagnose heart failure and monitor its status. Teach the patient why each test is being used and what he needs to do when the test is being conducted. Include these tests in your teaching, as indicated:
- electrocardiogram
- serum electrolyte levels

- arterial blood gas levels
- pulse oximetry
- chest X-ray, to determine heart and major vessel size. (X-rays also reveal the extent of pulmonary congestion.)

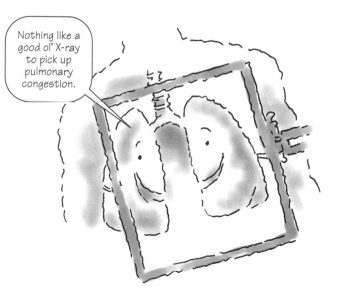

Teaching about activity and lifestyle

In the past, many patients with heart failure were advised to limit their activity. However, activity limitations are now indicated only for patients in the first stage of the disease. After initial recovery, patients should stay as active as possible.

Activity tips

Give your patient these activity tips:
- Pace yourself to avoid undue stress and fatigue.
- Follow your doctor's suggestions about activity and exercise, including sex.
- Practice deep-breathing, relaxation, and stress-relieving exercises.
- During rest periods, elevate your legs to prevent swelling.
- Wear antiembolism stockings during the day.
- Notify the doctor if activities seem to bring on shortness of breath, palpitations, or severe fatigue.

Zzzzzzzz...

To help your patient deal with possible sleep disturbances, cover these teaching points:

• If nocturia is a problem, help the patient adjust his diuretic schedule. For example, if he's taking a diuretic twice a day, advise him to take the second dose in the late afternoon or early evening.

• If orthopnea is a problem, suggest that the patient elevate the head of his bed on blocks or sleep in a recliner. Raising the head of the bed with blocks is more effective in maintaining airway patency than using several pillows when sleeping.

• If dyspnea awakens the patient shortly after he goes to bed, encourage him to elevate his feet for an hour before lying down. Explain that his shortness of breath may result from fluid in his legs returning to the main circulation. By elevating his feet before retiring for bed, he can prevent fluid accumulation in his lungs and allow his kidneys to clear excess fluid.

• Teach relaxation techniques to help the patient reduce his anxiety level.

• Because the patient may be more susceptible to respiratory infections, suggest

that he ask his doctor about pneumonia and influenza vaccines.
• Explain the need for regular medical check-ups.

Quick quiz

1. If your patient is anxious, teaching at that time may prove:
    A.   less effective.
    B.   more effective.
    C.   neither more nor less effective.
Answer: A. Anxiety and other emotional states increase the likelihood that teaching will be ineffective.

2. A low-sodium diet increases:
    A.   blood pressure.
    B.   cardiac workload.
    C.   urine output.
Answer: C. A low-sodium diet (2 to 3 g/day) increases urine output and prevents fluid accumulation.

3. Excellent sources of potassium include:

    A. legumes and poultry.
    B. dairy foods and dried fruits.
    C. green leafy vegetables and salmon.

Answer: C. Avocados, bananas, cantaloupes, carrots, dates, potatoes, green leafy vegetables, and salmon are all excellent sources of potassium.

4. Tell your patient to report a weight gain in 1 week of:

    A. 1 lb (0.45 kg).
    B. 2 lb (0.9 kg).
    C. 3 lb (1.35 kg).

Answer: C. Your patient should weigh himself daily, log each measurement in a diary, and report a weight gain of 3 lb (1.35 kg) or more in 1 week.

5. Dyspnea that awakens a patient shortly after he goes to bed may result from fluid:

    A. in his legs returning to the circulation.
    B. in his lungs being reabsorbed into blood vessels.
    C. in the sac surrounding the heart returning to the circulation.

Answer: A. Dyspnea that awakens a patient shortly after he goes to bed may result from fluid in his legs returning to the main circulation.

Scoring

☆☆☆   If you answered all five questions correctly, outstanding! You're our new Cardiac Teacher of the Year!

☆☆   If you answered four questions correctly, excellent! You're our new Cardiac Counselor of the Month!

☆   If you answered three or fewer questions correctly, take heart. We have a Cardiac Teaching Professional trophy right here, and it has your name on it!

Index

i refers to an illustration; t refers to a table.

i refers to an illustration; t refers to a table.

i refers to an illustration; t refers to a table.

i refers to an illustration; t refers to a table.

i refers to an illustration; t refers to a table.

i refers to an illustration; t refers to a table.

i refers to an illustration; t refers to a table.

i refers to an illustration; t refers to a table.

W

Weight
    desirable, 31t
    management of, 29-32, 31t, 123-124
    monitoring of, 47
World Wide Web, heart failure sites
        on, 125

X-Y

X-rays, chest, 68

Z

Zyban (bupropion), for smoking
        cessation, 34